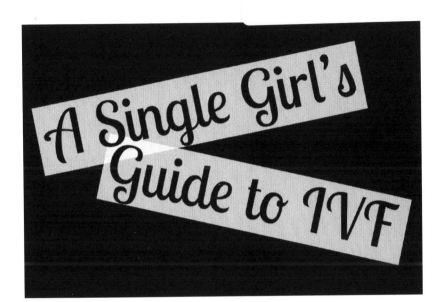

A Single Girl's Guide to IVF

Lisa Hoover
with Sarah Melland

ISBN: 978-0-6921-1403-2 (paperback)
ISBN: 978-0-6921-1425-4 (ebook)

Front Cover Design by: Sara Mason
www.saramason.wordpress.com

Note: The information in this book is true and complete to the best of our knowledge. This book is intended only as an informative guide for those wishing to know more about health issues. In no way is this book intended to replace, countermand, or conflict with the advice given to you by your own physician. The ultimate decision concerning care should be made between you and your doctor. We strongly recommend you follow his or her advice.

Dedicated to all the women going through infertility. And, yes, those are a smidgen of the 72 pregnancy tests I took on the cover.

Contents

Chapter 1
Single Mom by Choice

My name is Lisa Hoover. I'm "just a small-town girl living in lonely world" (Journey, 1981). I've fallen in love; I've fallen out of love. I've dated successful men; I've dated poor men. I've dated tall men; I've dated short men. I've dated the well-endowed, and I've dated baby carrots. I can always have men, but I can't always have a baby.

Dating in LA can be tiresome and draining. All the beautiful women competing with men of the same kind. All the fakers, takers, and filmmakers. It's hard to talk to men in bars. They already have their posses. Friends can be a good way to meet men, but it's trial and error. The only thing we're stuck with is online dating. It's not Wisconsin or Ohio, where people are ready to put down roots and start families in their early twenties. People in LA don't want to settle down. They want hustle and bustle. They want fame, fortune, and notoriety. Women want their careers and success before a family.

I moved to LA when I was eighteen to go to Loyola Marymount University for film and television production. I was wide-eyed and ambitious, and anything was possible. I could do anything in the land of dreams. At twenty-two, I formed a management company with my boyfriend Leo, whom I had met on the set of *Melrose Place* touring colleges in LA. Leo has charisma that lights up a room full of strangers. He's the life of the party—giving, caring, and a genuinely nice guy. He's the guy who buys shots for the whole bar. His heart is always bigger than his pocketbook.

Leo and I became best friends first and dated shortly after I transferred. Our company grew slowly, getting a few clients here and there. Nothing major, but enough to get by. By the time I was twenty-four, we had twenty-five clients actively working. My days were spent submitting clients for roles via casting notices, pitching clients to casting directors on the phone, and visiting sets when clients were working. It was never a job—it was fun.

My clients were family. We had movie nights, holiday parties, and gatherings at our condo in Beverly Hills. Our two bouncy chihuahuas were our kids. Leo would even secure them in a baby carrier when we browsed through the mall. Leo and I were inseparable—we lived together, worked together, and played together.

After a few more years, our relationship felt more like best friends than romantic partners. We had separate rooms but were still a family sharing money. Yes, a brother/sister relationship. Leo was my protective older brother, and when I say protective, I mean an overbearing, hovering helicopter mom. For years, everyone thought we were together. Although we weren't a couple anymore, we didn't step out on each other. When I was thirty-one, we got separate places, but we were still best friends, and we worked seamlessly together as our company hit all-time highs.

Leo got me a job working on *The Muppet Movie* with Jason Segel so I could get health insurance. Little did I know how much I would need it. Before Thanksgiving, during filming on the Warner Brothers back lot, I was struck by a canopy tent, immediately herniating two discs in my back and severing a nerve, causing cerebral spinal fluid to drain from my brain. This resulted in emergency surgery at Cedars-Sinai. Long story short: over the next five years, this resulted in five spinal surgeries, a spinal infection, enormous amounts of physical therapy, and a worker's comp case.

THE JOURNEY BEGINS

Back home in Ohio and recovering from my fifth back surgery, I am severely depressed. I am debilitated from having to step away from my prosperous talent management company, whose clients are thriving on movies like *The Fast and the Furious* and TV shows like *CSI: New York* and *Grey's Anatomy*.

Ohio at Christmas is right out of a Charles Dickens novel. Snow-covered trees, holiday decorations on houses, and lights on street poles. People greet you, and carolers stop by your door singing sweet melodies. It's a nice break from the harshness of LA. However, the weight gain and isolation from diminished social interaction takes a toll on my well-being. I'm alone for hours, lost in my thoughts. I wonder if this is it. These thoughts, along with the repetitive medical attention and physical pain, pull me into depression. I worry that it will always be this way. At some point, my negative thoughts get the better of me, and I seek help from a psychiatrist. I'm informed that physical pain and emotions run on the same neurotransmitters. When you feel continual physical pain, it can impact your emotions and stability. Oh, thank God. I thought I was crazy. Even George Clooney contemplated suicide after an agonizing spinal injury, stating, "I can't exist like this."

My sister has converted their three-car garage into a daycare facility, complete with its own kitchen. Their 3,500-square-foot house sits on nine acres with a pond and a barn. It's a daycare-meets-preschool, with vibrant colors, toys, and educational material. There are usually nine or ten children at a time, from newborns to four-year-olds.

I meet a bright, blue-eyed baby boy named Cooper. I'm put in charge of him exclusively, as he is only a month old and she's taking care of the older kids. Five days a week, ten hours a day, my focus is on keeping him safe. Cooper is a happy baby, a real snuggle bug. I always want to be near him, play with him, and hold him. Sometimes he sleeps on me for his naps. His smiles and coos warm my heart. I can't smother him enough with kisses. My love for him—a love I've never felt before—pulls me out of my depression. This experience makes me do a 180 on my opinion of children. In my twenties, I never wanted them. I'm content with my life, but young Cooper makes me realize there's something missing: the missing piece I didn't know was missing.

The thought of being a single mom by choice never crosses my mind until I have lunch with my high school girlfriend Michelle. Michelle is pretty, with shoulder-length brown hair and an athletic build. I haven't touched base with her since she married her wife.

We meet on a Tuesday. I'm weeping over a boyfriend who, of course, I think is the one. He, of course, doesn't.

"Get over it!" Michelle insists.

I don't want to get over it yet. I'm thirty-five and single, and my biological clock is ticking louder than a freight train passing by. I want the American dream. I want the horse-drawn carriage. I want a house I can't afford and a baby who has my flipping, flowing auburn locks. Is that too much to ask? I think not. It's not too much to ask. Not at all.

After a few minutes—maybe seven—of complaining about my farcical situation, Michelle stops me dead in my poorly paved tracks. "You don't need a man to have a baby. Do what I did: use a sperm donor." Ummm … yeah, right. No thank you. Sure, why don't I just go there right now? Hold my beer.

Who does that? Well, apparently everybody. Upwards of sixty thousand donor babies are born in America every year! I don't understand the concept of a sperm donor. For all I know, you walk into a sperm bank, and they hand you a random vial (vile!) from a dude who jacked off to a Nikki Benz porn. I don't want to end up with a middle-aged, balding, pot-bellied man in my tummy.

Michelle scolds me that I am being a stereotypical narcissist and proclaims it was the best decision of her life, as she has the cutest little boys. Her wife, Anne, carried their first child; Michelle carried their second; and eventually, Anne carried their third. They had bought enough sperm to each have two kids, with hopes of another in the future. They have a happy-go-lucky family and overfilled with joy.

I know if I want to do it the natural way, I'll have to meet a man, fall in love, get married (or not), and then be ready to start a family with him for life. That can potentially take years. I also don't want to rush a relationship with the wrong man, end up separated, then have his new bitch try to be my kid's baby mama. Not happening! Raising a kid by myself means no one can ever take them from me. 'Cause we all know how nasty custody battles can be. Since over half of marriages end in divorce, especially in LA (it's as high as 75 percent, no joke), I know my chances weren't swell.

I research adoption because I don't even need a baby. I would love to take an eight-year-old out of foster care. Each state has its own laws on adoption, but many adoptions are done through private agencies. They have their own regulations, which supersede state laws. Many include being married three to five years, long-term employment (meaning no self-employment), and no history of mental illness. Since I've been diagnosed with depression, my medical records will prevent adoption, and so will not being married and having my own company. Next time you tell someone they should just adopt, realize it's not that cut-and-dry. To this day, my friend Rich calls me selfish for wanting to bring a child into this world when there are many children who need families. Hey, Rich, guess what? My first thought was to adopt. It's unfortunate laws make it difficult for kids living in foster care with eight other kids in one bedroom who would love to have a single parent with their own space. I honestly just want to be a mom. Love makes a family, not DNA. I think about how much I love my fucking dogs, and they're canines. They don't share my DNA at all!

After two more months of thoroughly thinking about it (and not wanting to spend an astronomical fortune), I do the next best thing: I get hammered at a bar, searching for the ideal DNA my child is going to inherit—you know, the tall, dark, smart, witty, non-actor, handsome type who doesn't exist in LA. I end up with a short bodybuilder who wears a condom. Strike one. Waking up to his snoring, I think, *Shit, where's the nearest sperm bank?*

Chapter 2
The Not-So-Superior Sperm

It's the new year of 2015. Finally back in LA, unpacking my belongings in my quiet West Hollywood bungalow, I pour myself a sufficient glass of cabernet, something from Italy. I don't do well with wine from the US. I sit with my laptop and start my baby daddy search. I quickly come across the nation's largest sperm bank, California Cryobank, offering superior genetic material. I'm hooked. Ironically, it's based in LA, so I'm back to square one. Upside: most wannabe actors who are sperm donors have good bone structure.

I'm super excited to find they have more filters than a Brita. I have my own Brad Pitt at my fingertips. This cryobank specializes in celebrity doppelgangers. Let's get it done, Seth Rogen!

Here are just a few of the profiles I find on the California Cryobank website (https://cryobank.com/):

Donor 14340
LIGHTS, CAMERA, ACTION (FIGURES)

As a little boy, 14340 used to love playing with green army men. He would create elaborate detailed battle scenes and act them out. Although he may have outgrown the army men, his imagination hasn't faded a bit and he is now playing out his scenes from behind the camera—he's at school right now studying film (and sports medicine). While he considered entering business and law for money, he ultimately decided following his passion would make him happier and more fulfilled in life. He's already written one screenplay, loves watching films, and making short videos. When he's not busy calling "Action!" and "Cut!", he loves to play basketball and football and hang out with his friends, who say he's super loyal.

Donor Look-a-Likes
Josh Brolin (young), Josh Hartnett

DONOR 14868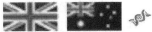
SIR LAUGH-A-LOT

The best thing about 14868 is his deep, hearty laugh. He laughs when he plays with his dog Brutus, sits in the audience at a comedy show, or swaps jokes with his best friends. He's great at making everyone feel at ease, and loves talking about crazy topics, whether it's nuclear energy, outer space, or Rubik's cubes. This patient, hardworking guy works as an engineer, and is fantastic at solving difficult problems with patience and ease. In his off time, this outdoorsman enjoys hiking, playing soccer with his brother, cooking, and defeating his friends in chess.

Donor Look-a-Likes:
Ashton Kutcher, Ben Barnes

Donor 15044
SWIMMING IN PSYCHOLOGY

This psychology major loves everything about neuroscience, but his true passions are on the beach! As the former president of his collegiate swim club, this veritable fish still teaches adult swim lessons after he gets off work. On the weekends, he plays volleyball in a national league, where his 6'3" stature certainly comes in handy! An adventurous spirit who loves the environment, 15044 buys only local produce, and has been known to take spontaneous bus trips to explore new cities.

Donor Look-a-Likes:
Sting (young), Liam Neeson

Donor 14893 **NEW**

CAPT. CREATIVE

14893's creativity knows no bounds. He paints, sculpts, dances, sings, and snaps photos. Even his body is a canvas featuring a couple of beautiful tattoos. This green-eyed guy definitely looks the part of an artist, sporting tousled brown hair, ever-changing facial hair styles, and faded t-shirts. Even though he loves making his own art, this vivacious, energetic teacher loves spreading his knowledge. In his free time, he teaches children how to make their own creations, and leads lessons with a booming voice of fun-loving attitude. In his free time, this outdoorsman loves to get away by camping, hiking, and kayaking.

Donor Look-a-Likes
Bradley Cooper, Wes Welker

Donor 14732

PhD MARTIAL ARTIST

This PhD candidate once fought in a cage match at a Mixed Martial Arts tournament in Bangkok. While he hung up his gloves years ago, this future epidemiologist claims his martial arts career prepared him for academia. If he can take a punch in front of screaming crowds, then he can certainly present research to a room of scientists! MMA career aside, this brainiac hopes to promote health and justice in the world, and is aiming for the top spot in his field.

Donor Look-a-Likes
Brandon Routh, Noah Bean

Donor 15202 **NEW**

PURSUIT OF HAPPINESS

Donor 15202 is an explorer and isn't afraid to throw caution to the side and give up a comfortable lifestyle to seek true happiness. On his own since 17, he believes that you should live in the moment and do what makes you happy. He isn't afraid to seek adventure; be it backpacking through Europe or quitting a corporate job that provided stability. Always eager to learn more about the world around him, this donor loves reading the encyclopedia. He believes that a person is truly tested when all they have is the clothes on their back. Using instincts to survive and passion to push through any life struggle, this donor is strong charismatic and thoughtful.

Donor Look-a-Likes
Casey Affleck, Rider Strong

I'm swiping right, swiping left, super liking, and adding to my favorites. How do you choose from this vast variety of unemployed aspiring actors and filmmakers? I can't help but feel slightly defeated, thinking, *Geez, I can't escape this pool of men.* I feel like I'm back to online dating, reading how these men like long walks on the beach and traveling to distant lands. I stop and take a minute. Even if I want it the natural way, no matter what, my baby is going to be an LA baby. *Stop being a dumbass, Lisa.*

Holy shit! Nine hundred and ninety-five dollars for a vial of creepy crawlers, plus $200 for shipping? Am I crazy? Soooo … my budget is just gonna go ahead and Google free options at the moment. Kaboom! Found my perfect match!

Once upon a time, when single women and infertile couples wanted a baby, they would pay a sperm bank. Sometimes it costs thousands of dollars for a successful pregnancy. But now, those services have gone online, and at the click of a mouse, donors make their sperm available by offering sex for free. A surprising—and some say unconventional—method of making a baby called "natural insemination."

CoParents.com is a social media platform aimed at providing a common ground to free sperm donors.

Simple Search!
All you need to do is register your personal needs and then browse through our comprehensive database of profiles.

Why Us?
At CoParents.com, we understand the human desire to born e a child and ensure our members are able to find suitable matches as per their prerequisites. With over 100,000 registrations, we have members from USA, UK, Australia … as well as Canada, and can safely say we are one of the most comprehensive databases of our kind.

Did I just hit bingo? A man is willing to have sex with me, I save money, and I get my baby? This could not go wrong. Don't worry, I'm only kidding. I don't do it, but this is a guide, and I'm letting you know all your options. "Natural insemination for the Tinder generation." If you want to look into sleeping with strangers/one-night stands, check out CoParents.com.

What is a girl to do? Is this worth it for me? Do I want to pay a thousand dollars for genetics I can't verify? Do I really, really want a baby? I think, *These websites only provide surface information and generic attributes. Am I too picky? I mean, this is permanent. If I'm going to spend a thousand dollars, I want to see what they will look like all grown up and not a picture at three years old. Everyone is cute as a baby.*

As I look around my empty room—an analogy to my life— I know this was going to be the right decision. I know I want a baby more than ever. The smiles, the cries, the ups, the downs, and the unconditional love I want to give.

As I sleep, I have the most vivid dream of me giving birth to a baby. I wake up in a hot sweat. I feel this soul is choosing me to be their parent. I can't sleep. I'm tossing and turning. I get out my laptop, and there, popping up on the sperm donor page, is Cooper, immediately calling me "Mama."

Alert

This donor currently has a **limited number of vials available.** Although more vials are expected to become avaliabe in the future, there is no guarentee that this will occur. Please consider this when selecting this donor.

To ensure continued vial availablilty, please take advantage of CCB's Family Today/Family Tomorrow Program. CCB Client Services is available at 866 927 9622 to answer any quesitons.

OK

In my sleep-deprived state, I impulsively buy five vials. I hope I remember this in the morning. I wake up feeling empowered. I got my donor; time to sew my wild oats one last time before I become preggo! All right, let's try this Tinder thingamajigger.

Chapter 3
The Last of the Booty Calls

My girlfriend encourages me to join Tinder. If you don't know what Tinder is, where have you been? It's a dating app leading people to one-night stands—maybe an occasional relationship, but highly unlikely. I put up a few selfies and write a brilliantly sophisticated profile. I'm not exactly sure how this app works, but some of these men are *forward*. I'm all for sex, but I need a little butter with my bread. "CUM OVR." Subtle. If only he'd spelled "over" correctly, I would have gone.

I get into a rhythm, swiping left. Oops, that guy looked hot. Stop! Swipe right. Oh, crap, wrong guy! I match with some dude named Kenny. Just my luck. Whatevs—I don't have to write back, but can they see if I read it? I won't read it. I'm such a rebel.

Twelve matches later, I go about my business and research fertility doctors. My phone is blowing up, and I find this kid, Noah (obvious name change for numerous reasons), who looks twenty-two. Great, I'm gonna rob the cradle—not the exact baby I wanted. I think, *Hey, what the hell? Young men have more stamina.* I like this decision already.

After way too much texting and a few dick pics, we decide to meet for Jack Daniels at his place. Don't worry, he sent me a pin of his place to my phone. Is this what millennials do? I thoroughly want some P in the V, and if I have to travel to do it, I have to travel to do it.

I walk down a dark street, texting my gf the address just in case I get killed. You can never be too careful. As the pin gets closer and closer, I get nervous butterflies in my system and have to convince myself this is what the younger generation does. He has never had a woman like me. I know what I'm doing. I'm ferocious; after all, I'm a Scorpio. I don't want a man screwing up my plan. I just want to screw a man or, in this case, a semi-man with a nice-sized peen (don't worry, he's 26). That's not bad. Men fornicate with women half their age; at least he isn't in the double digits.

He opens the door, shirtless, and what we have here is an Adonis. His body is astounding. His dark-brown hair, his chiseled six-pack with the deep V visible, and his piercing blue eyes penetrate my soul. *Good choice, Lisa. Thumbs up for you! Tinder gets an A. Where should I put my clothes? Where is the bedroom, or where would you like me?* This is all in my head, of course. What really happens is this take-charge boy throws me up against the door and kisses me. He leads me down the hall, and I ask to go to the restroom. Classy.

I put the toilet seat down and rest my head in my hands. *What am I doing? I can do this. People do this all the time. Girl, you are about to get inseminated, and you won't be having sex for nine months or potentially longer. This is your last hurrah. Get your shit together and take it like a champ.* I'm sweating like a banshee. I take some toilet paper and dab my armpits. I walk into his room and take off my boots. My zipper decides to jam. This is what I get for buying shoes online. His full-length mirrors want to make me keep my shirt on, but unfortunately, taking it off is the first thing he does. When he takes off his pants, I quickly realize he is *not* built like a white boy. Now I'm second-guessing my abilities. Oh, goodness gracious.

He slowly moves his way down my bosoms, licking every inch. Hair pulling, slapping, biting—nothing is off-limits. Roaring with excitement in copulation bliss, I tense my libido. I've been working on my Kegels, and I'm pleasantly impressed as he moans louder. The finale is equally as impressive as the appetizer.

Exactly what I needed. Time to leave like a boss. Not gonna lie: slightly upset I bought five vials of semen and just met the perfect gene sample. I casually dress, like he meant nothing to me. Nothing!

"So, I'll call you, but maybe not. We'll see." I struggle to get my jeans up my vivacious thighs.

Noah lights a joint, ignoring my cool comment. "All right."

"Yeah, I'm super busy."

"Cool."

"K. Bye."

"Yep."

I finally walk out. I'm ready to get this show on the road.

Chapter 4
Will You be My Donor?

It's been a month of researching doctors, hectic work schedules, and making appointments. Thank goodness LA is the mecca of fertility clinics. I'm able to get in right away. I'm filming a horror movie I'm producing with Leo. We dine at Fig, a nice poolside restaurant in Santa Monica, for a creative meeting. Palm trees, the ocean breeze, and the sun shining make this the perfect day for the exciting endeavor we are about to embark on.

Since LA is super ridiculously small, lo and behold, Noah stands in front of Leo and me with menus in his hand. Is this a sign? I'm about to meet with my fertility doctor, and Noah is staring me straight in the face. God, he's beautiful. Exotic. Underwear model. Dominator. As we stare deep into each other's eyes, Leo chimes in, "Are you going to seat us?"

Noah and I emerge from our trance. He brings us to a table. Leo sits as Noah leaves, "Who is that guy?" I don't want to talk to Leo about a sexcapade. I know his protective side. I'll get reprimanded for using Tinder and how dangerous it is.

"I've never met him before in my life."

Noah comes back around. "Sorry, it's my first day. I forgot to give you guys happy hour menus. You are looking good, Lisa."

15

Dead silence. Leo clasps his hands, places his elbows on table, and positions his body with authority. I slither down and hope I can slip under the table. Down, down, down I go.

"Get up here."

"No."

"Lisa, people are looking."

"I'm not telling."

"What. Did. You. Do?"

"I may have, or may not have, met him on a dating app."

"Which one?"

"Ummm—it's one of those where you swipe left or right."

"Tinder?"

"Something along those lines."

"Lisa, that's a hookup app."

"Oh, is it?" I put on my best dumb face. Leo stares intently. "It was just one night. Calm down!"

"*One night?!?* So, you *did* sleep with him?" Shit, I'm busted. "Do you know how dangerous that is?"

"I'm alive, aren't I? And look at how cute he is! Can you blame me?"

In an effort to keep this meeting short and sweet, I change the subject. "I brought you here to not only talk about the movie but also a pretty amazing personal idea I have come up with."

"What's that?"

"I'm going to have a baby."

"Oh my God, are you pregnant with that dude's baby?"

"No, I bought some sperm. I've done my research. I know what I am doing."

"Oh, you have a donor already? What's he like?"

"Eh, a donor. Above par, probably."

"Well, why don't you just shoot for the top and ask Tinderboy over there?" I ponder this for a moment. I already think he looks spectacular as either a boy or a girl.

"That might actually work." I'm impressed with this idea.

"I'm joking."

"I'm not. I want the best. I mean, he's working as a host. He must need the money."

"Wait, what? You would pay him?"

"It's only fair. A so-so vial of genes runs a grand. Why not pay to get exactly what I want?"

"Lisa, this is one of the most harebrained ideas I have ever heard."

"No, I am dead serious. Don't look at me that way. How can I use this as a bargaining chip? Also, how do I ask him?"

"I am not participating in this conversation any longer."

I anxiously try to figure out the words to ask Noah to be my sperm donor. How am I going to ask a random dude to be my baby backer? I'm knocking my knuckles on the table. My legs are crossed, and my foot is moving back and forth. I can do this. This kid stands to make four grand. I mean, who wouldn't want to do that, just to jack off in a cup, right? That is such easy money.

I text Noah to meet me for dinner. He agrees. At the bar, he rubs my leg, but I pull away and take a huge gulp of my drink.

"Is everything okay? Isn't this, like, our arrangement? Or do you have another fantasy I can fulfill?"

I laugh coyly. *If you only knew what I am about to ask you.* I slap his leg playfully.

"No, silly. What's new with you? It's been ages." Noah looks at me, not understanding the words coming out of my mouth.

"I don't think we have ever had a real conversation."

"Well, why not start now?" I smile. "Are you going to college? An actor? Have you ever had a debilitating disease, maybe a heart palpitation?"

"Not that I know of. Definitely not an actor. That shit is so superficial. No offense."

"None taken. I hate actors. I just represent them."

"I'm studying law at USC." This kid keeps getting better and better.

"You want to be a lawyer?"

"Yeah, something like that. We're not having sex tonight, are we?" *Oh, man, just ask him. Say you have a business proposition for him. Simple. Easy. Direct.*

"No."

"Okay. Well, I'm gonna go." *Of course you would. You're nine years younger than me. Why wouldn't you go and get some pootie tang every night?*

So what? I chickened out. I'll just ask via text. Everyone asks life-changing questions via text. I mean, it *is* 2016. Also, you can hide behind text messages. I don't have to see the look on his face.

Once again, my internal dialogue runs rampant. *This isn't crazy. This is business. Business as usual. A great business opportunity. Business. Business. Business? Oh, mother Mary. Here goes nothing.*

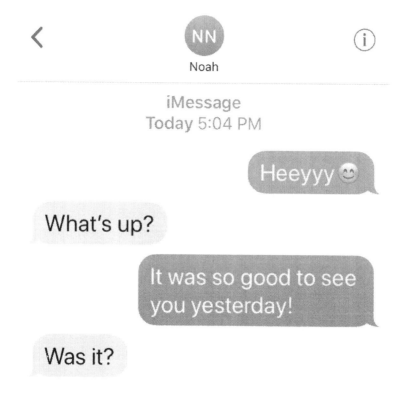

Yeah. Quick question. Soooo....have you ever thought of being a sperm donor?

Huh?

Yeah, like for money.

Oh, like a sperm bank?

Uh-huh

Yeah. When I was an undergrad me and my frat brothers thought about doing it for extra cash.

Would you consider doing it now?

It doesn't pay that much.

Well, what if it did?

What's up with this line of questioning?

(Inner monologue: *Let the word "vomit" proceed.*)

No one really knows, but I want to be a mom and I don't want to wait for a man to do it. I looked into sperm banks and haven't found the right donor. Then I met you and thought wow! He would make a pretty baby. Once I got to know you, I found you have a lot of great attributes to pass along to a child.

Thanks?

(Inner monologue: *Quick, think of something. You're losing him! Remember the money. He's a poor college student.*)

Those guys only get $150 a sample but they sell for a $1,000. I'd be willing to give you the $1,000 if you are willing to help me. Help me, help you.

I don't know. Donating to a sperm bank I won't know the kids, but with you, I know you. That's weird.

People do it all the time. It's fine. You don't know me.

You're right. I don't know you. This is a lot to ask. I have to think about it.

  iMessage

Noah joins me at Frolic Room in Hollywood to discuss the arrangement. The walls are plastered with caricatures of actors from Hollywood's Golden Era. The dimly lit setting is perfect for an intimate conversation.

"So, have you thought about it?" Noah chokes on his drink. "*Oh*, you were serious?"

"What are you doing this weekend? I have $500." I know I'm ovulating. Try it the natural way first and save ass-tons of money.

"So, what? You want me to go to a doctor's office?"

"No, I want to have sex, idiot. Is that a problem?"

"I don't know if I'm comfortable doing it that way, since it really does seem like I'm creating my own child."

"Do you feel like that every time you have sex with women?" *Inappropriate, Lisa. Save yourself.* "Listen, it will be quick, easy, and fun. We've done it before. This time, cum inside."

"I don't know if I'm ready to be a dad."

"I'm not asking you to be a dad. I'm asking you to relinquish your parental rights. I don't want you, only your heredity."

"Oh. So can we do a contract?"

"Yes. What would you want me to put in it? I'll draw one up with my lawyer."

"Look, I got a social life and school to worry about. I really don't want anyone to know it's me."

"Sure."

After a lot of talking and a lot more wine, we agree to all the terms. This is my actual sperm donor agreement. You only have to do this when the donor is known; if it comes from a sperm bank, the donor has already relinquished his parental rights, and the paperwork is done by the facility.

This agreement is necessary to address both parties' needs and concerns in an up-front, honest manner. For me, it's about him relinquishing all parental rights, and for him, it's about being released from any financial or physical responsibility. Terms are outlined, including payment and terms required. It's best to be on the same page before you proceed with the donor.

DONOR AGREEMENT

This agreement is made this 1ˢᵗ day of March 2016 by and between Noah Noname, hereafter referred to as the DONOR, and Lisa Hoover, hereafter referred to as the RECIPIENT, who may be collectively referred to as "Parties."

NOW, THEREFORE, in consideration of the promises of each other, DONOR and RECIPIENT agree as follows:

1. Each clause of the AGREEMENT is separate and divisible of each other, and should a court refuse to enforce one or more clauses of the AGREEMENT, the others are still valid and in full force.
2. The DONOR has agreed to provide his semen to the RECIPIENT for the purpose of insemination.
3. In exchange for the DONOR's services, the RECIPIENT agrees to pay the sum of $1,000 to the DONOR for two semen donations per cycle (25 days).
4. Each Party is single and has never been married.
5. Each Party acknowledges and agrees during the calendar year of 2016, the RECIPIENT is attempting to become pregnant by insemination and such inseminations will continue until conception occurs.
6. If conception occurs before commencement of 2016, RECIPIENT agrees to pay DONOR for remaining cycles in which donations did NOT occur.
7. Each Party agrees the DONOR is providing his semen for the purpose of said insemination and does so with the clear understanding he will not demand, request, or compel any guardianship or custody of the child(ren) resulting from the insemination. Further, the DONOR acknowledges he will have no parental rights whatsoever with the child(ren).
   a. RECIPIENT agrees to allow DONOR visitation with the child(ren) when requested.
   b. In the event of RECIPIENT's death, DONOR will be reinstated his parental rights, including guardianship and custody of child(ren). If DONOR does not wish to have these rights or responsibilities, DONOR agrees to transfer custody of child(ren) to person(s) stated in RECIPIENT's Will.
8. Each Party acknowledges the sole authority to name any child(ren) resulting from the insemination shall rest with the RECIPIENT.
9. Each Party acknowledges and agrees the Natural Insemination used to receive the semen donations, as well as the execution of the AGREEMENT, were specifically chosen to avoid any finding that the DONOR is a legal father to the child(ren) pursuant to California AB 960. Consistent with that purpose, each Party has executed this AGREEMENT with the purpose of clarifying her or his intent to release and relinquish any and all rights she or he may have to bring a suit to establish paternity of any child(ren) conceived through insemination.

10. Each Party acknowledges and agrees the DONOR shall not be held responsible for legal, financial, medical, or emotional needs of said child(ren).

11. Each Party covenants and agrees that, in light of the exceptions of each Party, as stated above, RECIPIENT shall have absolute authority and power to appoint a guardian for her child(ren) and the RECIPIENT and such guardian may act with sole discretion as to all legal, financial, medical, and emotional needs of said child(ren) without any involvement or demands of authority from DONOR.

12. Each Party covenants and agrees none of them will identify the DONOR as the parent of the child(ren), nor will either of them reveal the identity of the DONOR to any of their respective relatives or to any individuals without the express written consent of the other Party.

13. Each Party acknowledges and agrees relinquishment of all rights, as stated above, is final and irrevocable. The DONOR further understands his waivers shall prohibit action on his part for custody or guardianship EXCEPT in the event of the case of the RECIPIENT'S death.

14. Each Party acknowledges and agrees any future contact with the DONOR with any child(ren) that result from the insemination in no way alters the effect of this agreement. Any such contact will be at the sole discretion of the RECIPIENT and will be consistent with the intent of both Parties to sever all parental rights and responsibilities of the DONOR. All Parties do also acknowledge that in the best interest of the child(ren), if the child(ren) at any time requests to meet or form a friendship with the DONOR, it is the intention of the DONOR to be receptive to such contact. All agree any friendship formed between the DONOR and the child(ren) does not construe a parental relationship with any of its concomitant rights or responsibilities.

15. The DONOR agrees to keep the RECIPIENT updated with current address and contact information so that the child(ren) can make contact in the future.
    a. DONOR agrees to be available for two meetings during consecutive days of fertility window during RECIPIENT's ovulation. RECIPIENT agrees to give DONOR knowledge of such meeting dates each cycle at her earliest knowledge.
    b. Each Party agrees to be available to each other via text message, email, and phone calls.
    c. Each Party maintains they are STD and HIV negative and will continue safer sex practices during this arrangement.

16. Each Party covenants and agrees any dispute pertaining to the AGREEMENT that arises between them shall be subject to the following process:
    a. Step 1: Family Counselor Session
    b. Step 2: Mediator
    c. Step 3: Binding Arbitrations

       i. Family counselor and arbitration team will be chosen and agreed upon by both Parties. Costs of the above processes shall be divided equally by both Parties.

17. Each Party acknowledges and understands there may be legal questions raised by the issues involved in this AGREEMENT which have not been settled by statute or prior court decision. Notwithstanding the knowledge that certain clauses stated herein may not be enforced by a court of law, the Parties choose to enter into this AGREEMENT and understand the meaning and significance of each provision of the AGREEMENT.

18. Each Party acknowledges and agrees she or he signed this AGREEMENT voluntarily and freely by his or her own choice, without any duress of any kind whatsoever. It is further acknowledged each Party has had the time to review this AGREEMENT and understands the meaning of significance of each provision of the AGREEMENT.

19. Each Party acknowledges and agrees any changes made in the terms and conditions of the AGREEMENT shall be made in writing and signed by both Parties.

20. This AGREEMENT contains the entire understanding of the Parties. There are no promises, understandings, agreements, or representations between the Parties other than those expressly stated in this AGREEMENT. In witness whereof, the Parties hereunto have executed this AGREEMENT, consisting of two typewritten pages, in the City of Los Angeles, County of Los Angeles, State of California, on the date and the year first written above.

You are welcome for the free contract I had to pay $500 for. Love you guys. And you are welcome for its being only two and a half pages, ten-point font.

Noah and I meet at a random Chase bank in Venice to get the contract signed and notarized.

The notary reads the contract. He looks at us like we're effing nuts. "Do you have a problem with this arrangement?" I lash out.

"No, no, just something I've never seen before." We sign the contract in front of him. He copies our licenses, then stamps the contract. Signed, sealed, and delivered.

Chapter 5
Bring on the Professionals

On the day of my reproductive endocrinologist appointment, I am over-the-moon ecstatic. I am going to do this. I am going to be a mom. This is where I am going to be real with you. I thought I would be pregnant in a couple months max; as far as I knew, nothing was wrong with me. I just never tried to get pregnant. If I had I known going into it that I had a two-year journey ahead of me, I don't know if I would have put myself through it. Optimism is the fuel to getting through infertility.

I am let down by the sterile doctor's office. I had pictured an office with baby announcements and grateful letters from new parents posted on the walls. This is not it. This is clinical and cold. I sign in and fill out paperwork for a new patient. I sit and wait. And wait. And wait. Check my phone and wait some more. See a pamphlet of all the different fertility treatments and decide to indulge myself in what I might have to embark on.

FERTILITY DRUGS/PMS INDUCERS
The Lowdown: Injected or taken in pill form, the drugs release hormones inducing ovulation to boost egg production and makes the uterus more receptive to embryo implantation.

The Candidates: Women who don't ovulate regularly or who have partners with very poor sperm quality. Avoid if you have damaged, blocked fallopian tubes or scarring from endometriosis.

The Chances: Forty to forty-five percent of women who take the pills and ovulate get pregnant. Fifty percent of women who ovulate as a result of the shots get pregnant.

The Good: Typically, the first choice in fertility treatment because of low cost and relative convenience.

The Bad: Possible bloating, headaches, hot flashes, and nausea. Side effects are worse with the shots and include risk of multiple births, premature delivery, and formation of large ovarian cysts.

The Ugly: Varies widely. For example, from $60–$6,000 per cycle. Like I said, widely.

ARTIFICIAL INSEMINATION
(INTRAUTERINE INSEMINATION OR IUI)

The Lowdown: Specially prepared washed* sperm is inserted directly into the uterus through a thin, flexible catheter during IUI. If you choose this method, your doctor might recommend you take fertility drugs to increase the chances of fertilization.

*Washed sperm is where the embryologist separates sperm from the semen. They remove chemicals from the semen that may cause adverse reactions in the uterus.

The Candidates: Men with slow-moving or lower-quality sperm or a low sperm count; women who have produced antibodies to their partner's sperm or whose cervical mucus (CM) is too scant, acidic, or thick to transport the sperm to the egg.

The Chances: Depends on a woman's age and the quality of the man's sperm. In general, there's a 15–20 percent chance of conception per cycle, with a 60–70 percent chance of pregnancy after six cycles. It's a mathematical estimate of your odds—each cycle in and of itself, meaning it doesn't get better each cycle. You like to gamble? It's the Russian roulette of pregnancy. Do you feel lucky? Well, do ya, punk?

The Good: A simple procedure performed in a doctor's office.

The Bad: Can result in multiple births; possible side effects of fertility drugs.

The Ugly: On average, $865 per cycle.

DONOR SPERM

The Lowdown: Sperm from a man other than the intended father is used during IUI or IVF.

The Candidates: Couples experiencing male factor infertility; men carrying genetic disorders they don't want to pass on to their children; single women; or lesbian couples.

The Chances: An estimated 15 percent of women who try this method get pregnant after one cycle, with up to 80 percent achieving pregnancy after six cycles. Again, with mathematics. I hope you studied. There will be an exam after.

The Good: Enables infertile men, carriers of genetic disorders, and single or lesbian women to have a child.

The Bad: Some men might be uncomfortable with a donor who has no genetic relationship to them. You also don't get to see what these half-wits look like all grown up. Just saying.

The Ugly: $700–$1,000 per cycle, generally. Factors that may affect the cost include whether you want a donor consultation and photo match, need storage for the sperm, or want washed sperm.

IN VITRO FERTILIZATION (IVF)

The Lowdown: Multistep process (called a cycle) in which your eggs are extracted and fertilized with sperm in a lab. Once embryos develop, one or two are implanted in your uterus, and the rest are stored.

The Candidates: Older women; women with blocked or severely damaged fallopian tubes or scarring from endometriosis; men with poor sperm quality; couples with unexplained infertility.

The Chances: Varies by age and doctor. Forty-one percent of women under age thirty-five, 32 percent of women between ages 35–37, and 23 percent of women between ages 38–40 become pregnant.

The Good: Couples with serious fertility problems can become parents.

The Bad: Treatments are costly, physically demanding, and require a rigorous regimen of fertility drugs before the start of each cycle.

The Ugly: $8,000, on average, per cycle, not including medications.

INTRACYTOPLASMIC SPERM INJECTION (ICSI)

The Lowdown: An embryologist selects a healthy-looking single sperm from the male's semen and injects it directly into the egg with a microscopic needle. Once an embryo develops, it's transferred into the uterus through IVF.

The Candidates: Men with very low sperm count or poor sperm quality.

The Chances: About 35 percent of those undergoing ICIS with IVF will become pregnant.

The Good: Men who have a very low sperm count can become biological fathers.

The Bad: Costly and involved procedure; the drugs required for IVF have many side effects.

The Ugly: $1,000–$2,000 per cycle, excluding the cost of IVF.

DONOR EGGS

The Lowdown: Eggs obtained from the ovaries of another woman (usually younger) are fertilized by sperm from the recipient's partner. Resulting embryos are then transferred into the recipient's uterus.

The Candidate: Women whose ovaries are damaged or prematurely failing or who have undergone chemotherapy and/or radiation; older women with poor egg quality; and women carrying genetic disorders they don't want to pass along.

The Chances: Fifty-five percent of women using fresh donor eggs* will give birth; the number drops to 34 percent for frozen eggs. **

*Fresh eggs are when a donor cycles exclusively for you. Donor eggs are retrieved and immediately fertilized by the sperm. Frozen eggs are from a woman who previously did a cycle and are frozen. Eggs have to be thawed in order to fertilize; not all eggs will thaw properly.

**Frozen eggs should *never* be shipped, as freezing protocols differ from lab to lab. These differences can cause a breakdown of egg quality when thawed. If you plan to use frozen eggs, use donors whose eggs are stored in-house with the fertility clinic. Either use frozen eggs already at your lab or pay the extra money for fresh eggs. It makes a huge difference.

The Good: Enables older women and those with ovarian problems to become mothers.

The Bad: The procedure is expensive; the recipient must take a rigorous drug regimen with many potential side effects. Some women with no genetic link to the donor eggs may be uncomfortable using them.

The Ugly: $20,000 (the cheapest when using frozen eggs) to $50,000 (a guaranteed cycle, meaning guaranteed baby or money back); includes IVF and compensation for the donor.

SURROGACY

The Lowdown: The surrogate becomes pregnant by artificial insemination using the father's sperm or through IVF with the couple's embryo. Donor eggs and sperm may also be used.

The Candidates: Women who can't carry a baby because of disease, hysterectomy, or infertility. In rare instances, both partners are infertile.

The Chances: Depends on the quality of the eggs and sperm being used. On average, though, live birth rates range from 5–30 percent per cycle.

The Good: Can help couples with fertility issues such as what happened to Kim Kardashian, which was preeclampsia and placenta accrete.* Women who don't have a uterus or who have a disease preventing pregnancy can become parents.

*Placenta accrete: The placenta grows so deeply into the uterus that it cannot be separated after delivery. In severe cases, it can grow completely through the uterus and even reach the bladder or other organs. Often the treatment is the removal of the uterus at the time of the delivery. Even in cases where the uterus can be saved, the uterus may have significant scarring or otherwise be unable to carry a pregnancy.

The Bad: Costs are prohibitive. Couples may feel removed from the pregnancy and have to deal with an array of state surrogacy laws and legal contracts.

The Ugly: Between $50,000 and $100,000, depending on issues like whether IVF is needed, fees to the surrogate agency, and compensation for the surrogate mom.

DONOR EMBRYOS

The Lowdown: Embryos are donated by couples undergoing IVF who become pregnant and no longer need unused fertilized eggs. The donated embryo is transferred into the recipient. This is an alternative to adoption and also an option for women who want to experience bearing a life. There are religious organizations that object to discarding embryos (believing life begins at conception) and do embryo adoptions. The big agency is called Snowflake Embryo Adoption by Nightlight Christian Adoptions (www.nightlight.org). Give birth to your own adopted baby.

The Candidates: Couples in which both woman and man are infertile but want to experience a pregnancy.

The Chances: The live birth rate is about 30–50 percent, depending on how many embryos are implanted and whether they are fresh or frozen. (See above for description, in case you forgot.)

The Good: Enables infertile couples to have a childbearing experience.

The Bad: Medical screening, a rigorous fertility drug regimen, and lots of legalities. It may be hard to find donated embryos, as couples might be reluctant to give their "technical" offspring up.

The Ugly: $15,000–$30,000 per cycle; again, depends on fresh or frozen.

REPRODUCTIVE SURGERY

The Lowdown: Surgery—sometimes requiring a hospital stay, sometimes done on an outpatient basis—is used to correct anatomical abnormalities, remove scarring, and clear blockages in either the man or the woman.

The Candidates: Couples with diagnosed diseases or abnormalities.

The Chances: Depends largely on the condition, severity, and one's age. In one study, women who were treated laparoscopically for endometriosis had about double the pregnancy rate of those who were not treated.

The Good: Besides reducing pain or discomfort associated with the disease, it may increase the likelihood of pregnancy.

The Bad: Some surgeries are more invasive than others, which can increase the risk, cost, and recovery time.

The Ugly: Depends on the surgery, the surgeon, and what's involved. Laparoscopic surgery for endometriosis can cost anywhere from $1,700 to $5,000.

GAMETE INTRAFALLOPIAN TRANSFER (GIFT)

The Lowdown: Eggs from the woman are collected, mixed with sperm from the man in a petri dish, and placed directly inside the fallopian tubes, where fertilization can occur. You still have to do your own magic because the eggs aren't fertilized yet. Fingers crossed.

The Candidates: Couples in which the woman has at least one functioning fallopian tube and/or the man has a low sperm count or sperm with poor motility; couples who have unexplained infertility.

The Chances: Twenty-five to thirty percent of GIFT cycles will result in pregnancy; younger, healthier women have a higher success rate.

The Good: Allows fertilization to occur in a natural environment.

The Bad: No immediate verification fertilization has occurred. A more complicated procedure than IVF because a laparoscope is used to insert the egg/sperm mix into the tubes. If more than one egg is used (and it typically is), there is a higher-than-normal risk of multiple births.

The Ugly: $15,000–$20,000 per cycle.

ZYGOTE INTRAFALLOPIAN TRANSFER (ZIFT)

The Lowdown: Like IVF, but in this case, the embryo is inserted into the fallopian tube, not the uterus. The minute an egg is fertilized, it's called a zygote. It is twenty-four hours after fertilization instead of a day 3 morula or day 5 blastocyst into the uterus. It spends more time in the body than the lab. Some people feel the body is a better incubator than a petri dish.

The Candidates: Couples who have unexplained infertility or men with low sperm count; the woman has at least one tube open; and/or there are ovulation problems.

The Chances: Depends on age and health. In general, 36 percent of couples using ZIFT become pregnant during a cycle, with 29 percent going on to deliver.

The Good: Fertilization of the egg/sperm mixture, now called a zygote, can be confirmed before placed into the fallopian tube (not the case with GIFT). Therefore, fewer eggs may be used, lowering the risk of a multiple birth.

The Bad: Because a laparoscope is used, it is considered invasive surgery, increasing risks and costs compared to IVF. GIFT and ZIFT are rarely used.

The Ugly: $8,000–$13,000 per cycle.

If you aren't deterred by any of this, you are a perfect candidate. For some odd reason, this doesn't shock me. The nurse finally calls me. She checks my blood pressure and, of course, they take my weight. I always hate that. Let me take off my shoes first, and please deduct ten pounds for my clothes.

Since this is not going to be a positive doctor review, he will remain Dr. Nameless, because I'm still not sure if I should sue his ass. You'll see. I'll explain later. This is why I'm writing this book: so you don't have to go through the hell I did.

I sit in the office with Dr. Nameless and his equally unnamed med student. The reason I'm mentioning the med student is because he was hot, hot, hot, and it killed me. He always did my vaginal exams. If you have a doctor with a med student, don't hesitate to ask the doctor to do the exams; it will be a lot less painful. Sorry, med student, you have not picked up the finesse yet.

After the generic "Tell me about yourself" questions, I begin to explain my situation. I explain I want to be a single mom. I want to venture having a child, and I have a donor. The doctor asks which cryobank I use, assuming I want to do an IUI.

"Oh, no sir. I know him."

"Great. So we are going to do an IUI?"

"Again, no. I was thinking we could do organic insemination."

"Excuse me?"

The med student chimes in with his two cents, proclaiming, "She wants to have sex with him."

I smile. "Correct."

"Well, you need to hire an attorney and get a contract together."

"Already done." He oversteps his bounds by asking for the lawyer's name and a copy of the signed contract. That's really none of his business.

He orders an array of blood tests and genetic testing. Being naïve and new, I don't ask questions. I assume everything is okay. From past history with doctors, no news is good news, am I right? Or confused? I'll go with I'm right but probably confused.

Chapter 6
Medicated

Enthusiastic, eager, and with prescription in hand, I will make a baby this month. Dr. Nameless put me on a low dose of 50 mg of Clomid to start on the third day of my period. I continue through day 7.

I have my first ultrasound to check my follicle sizes. A follicle is a fluid-filled sac containing an immature egg. During ovulation, a mature egg is released from a follicle. While several follicles begin to develop each cycle, normally only one will ovulate an egg. Things are going well; I have two mature follicles on one side and one on the other. The doctor says I am ready to take my trigger shot. A trigger shot is a medication of human chorionic gonadotropin (hCG) that induces ovulation (the release of eggs from the ovary).

I inject myself with Ovidrel, prompting the release of all my mature eggs within 24–36 hours. I've been given exact times to schedule procreation. Well, that's not ideal. Noah is infamously late. Why can't he ever come (cum) on time? Lame single-girl joke.

Although I only took two medications this cycle, there's an overabundance of fertility drugs used in different treatments. Little did I know what I was in for. Saying this with a bit of a laugh.

ALL OF THE MEDS

The costs listed for these drugs are cash prices. Most insurance doesn't cover fertility treatments or medication.

BRAVELLE/FERTINEX/FOLLISTIM/GONAL-F/METRODIN (Follicle-Stimulating Hormone)
SEROPHENE/CLOMID
(Clomiphene Citrate—Same as above)

The Good: They trick your body into thinking it's in menopause. It increases your follicle-stimulating hormone (FSH) in order to produce more eggs in the ovaries.

The Bad: Upset stomach, bloating, abdominal fullness, hot flashes, breast tenderness, headaches, dizziness. Can cause mental and mood changes. It's nicknamed CloMAD because people often get angry when they take it.

The Ugly: $25–$100, depending on IUIs.

The Truth: Welcome to your amped-up PMS cycle. Get ready to be an emotionally unstable, crying bitch. I'm looking at my aquarium, admiring the fish, when I see three of the mollies playing on one side of the tank and one by itself in the corner. I bawl. They are ostracizing that one fish. I'm genuinely upset. My heart feels for the tiny fish. I know it's ridiculous.

During my next beautiful transition on Clomid, I'm at the iconic Beverly Center mall, wearing short sleeves in the middle of our LA winter. Bath & Body Works is having a sale on three-wick candles. The sales associate tries to help me find more pumpkin scents when my face starts to flush. Legit sweat running down my face. The sales girl trembles. "Are you ok?"

"I can't breathe. Is it hot in here?" Desperate to find water, I run to locate a stupid vending machine, since the food court is never close. I push an adolescent out of the way and guzzle a Dasani, pouring it all over my face like I'm in a Cindy Crawford

Pepsi commercial. If I could, I'd rip my clothes off here and now. Just going to put it right here: Clomid is the worst for me.

CETROTIDE/GANIRELIX ACETATE
(Gonadotropin-Releasing Hormone Antagonist)

The Good: Stops eggs from being released too early and gives eggs time to grow properly. This medication blocks release of luteinizing hormone (LH). The rise of LH triggers ovulation. When you use ovulation predictor kits, they turn positive when a surge of LH is in your urine.

The Bad: Pain, bruising, redness, swelling, itching at the injection site, nausea, and headaches.

The Ugly: $200–$400, depending on dose.

The Truth: I was getting headaches even after I received my Botox treatment (obviously for medical purposes, but not really, but maybe).

CRINONE/PROMETRIUM
(Progesterone)

The Good: Increases thickness of uterine lining. Helps with receiving a fertilized egg and implantation. Also needed to maintain pregnancy.

The Bad: Stimulates side effects that look like pregnancy. A lot of women get tricked into thinking they are pregnant when they are not. Bloating, cramps, stomach pain, constipation, diarrhea, nausea, breast swelling and pain, pain around the vaginal area, drowsiness, tiredness, decreased interest in sex, joint pain, headaches.

The Ugly: $15 for one 8 percent tube of Crinone. $350 for 100 capsules of Prometrium. $1–$3 per pill of progesterone; up to $7 per insert. $50 for a vial of progesterone in oil.

The Truth: Doesn't all this medicine sound amazing? Get ready to invest in a big box of pantiliners because the discharge will make you feel like you're peeing yourself 24/7. I'm tired of pantiliners. The other option is progesterone in oil, which comes with a huge fucking needle and requires daily injections in your ass muscle. It causes bruising, soreness, and muscle aches. Yeah, it's tough to decide which one to choose, I know. I feel you. It's hard.

DOSTINEX/PARLODEL
(Prolactin Reducing)

The Good: Prolactin is made in your pituitary gland and stimulates the production of breast milk. So if you have high levels of prolactin in your body, this reduces it, as your body might think it's pregnant.

The Bad: Nausea, vomiting, upset stomach, constipation, dizziness, light-headedness, tiredness.

The Ugly: $250 for 8.5 mg tablets of Dostinex. $75 for 30 2.5 mg tablets of Parlodel.

The Truth: I'm sure you have already guessed what amazing side effect this has. Get ready to leak milk, bitches! Upside: it increases your libido, gives a mood boost, and "really doubles the pleasure." Dammit, I wish I had had a man during that period.

Side note: women peak sexually in their thirties.

FACTREL/LUTREPULSE
(Gonadotropin-Releasing Hormone)

The Good: Used by women who are missing menstrual periods. Provides GNH the body needs for growth and release of mature eggs from the ovaries. Mature follicles measure over 16 mm.

The Bad: Headache, nausea, abdominal pain with menstrual bleeding, skin rash.

The Ugly: $25 for a vial of Factrel. $175 for a vial of Lutrepulse.

The Truth: I never took this one, but it doesn't sound too bad. No mood swings seem like a plus, and the skin rash sounds appealing.

FEMARA
(Letrozole)

The Good: Like Clomid, different compounds used to treat infertile women who need assistance to ovulate. (FDA approved for use as a breast cancer drug, used off label for fertility treatments.)

The Bad: Fatigue, dizziness, headache, bloating, hot flashes, night sweats, blurred vision, upset stomach, breast pain, difficulty sleeping, spotting, or unusual menstrual bleeding.

The Ugly: $325 for 32.5 mg tablets; thirty-day supply.

The Truth: Again, different compound, same results. See Clomid.

HUMEGON/MENOPUR/PERGONAL/REPRONEX
(Human Menopausal Gonadotropin)

The Good: Provides FSH and LH, which help healthy ovaries make eggs.

The Bad: Headaches, stomachaches, bloating, redness/pain at the injection site, breast tenderness, and dizziness.

The Ugly: $85 for a vial of Menopur, $10 for a vial of Humegon (sounds little, but you will need multiple vials), $72 for a vial of Pergonal, $36 for a vial of Repronex.

The Truth: This drug is taken in combination with other drugs on a stimulating cycle. A stimulating cycle is a period of time when fertility drugs are used for ovarian stimulation to mature multiple eggs in a single cycle. This makes it hard to tell which side effects are coming from which medicine. I would just like to say they all make you equally nuts.

My whole goal was to find a space on my stomach sans bruising. When I did, it was a gold star day. I'm an expert with my needle-stabbing skills. I would do a Picasso on my stomach—an epic painting of black, blue, and yellow hues washing over a sea of flesh.

LUPRON
(Leuprolide Acetate)

The Good: Mainly used to treat men with symptoms of prostate cancer. Used in women to treat symptoms of endometriosis.

The Bad: A nice array of headaches, hot flashes, increased sweating, night sweats, tiredness, upset stomach, nausea, and redness/burning/stinging/pain/bruising at the injection site.

The Ugly: $568 for a two-week supply.

The Truth: I used this in a frozen embryo transfer (FET) cycle. It suppresses the pituitary gland to decrease the chance of ovulation occurring unexpectedly. All these drugs prep my lining to receive the embryo. The last thing they want is to ovulate and ruin the cycle. These caused mad headaches—like, I'm talking a twenty-four-hour migraine with a wet washcloth on your forehead. #NoJoke #NotExaggerating #Horrible #Miserable #Debilitating

NOVAREL/OVIDREL/PREGNYL/PROFASI
(HUMAN CHORIONIC GONADOTROPIN)

The Good: The hCG shots are used to trigger ovulation. Ovulation should happen within 24–36 hours after injection. Used during IUIs and IVFs to properly schedule the time for insemination and egg retrievals.

The Bad: Nausea, vomiting, abdominal pain/swelling, headache, restlessness, irritability, water weight gain, depression.

The Ugly: $300 for a vial, depending on size, of Novarel. $170 for .5 ml (starts to laugh) of Ovidrel, $100 for 10,000 units (may sound like a lot, but it's a small vial) of Pregnyl.

The Truth: Can you imagine taking multiples of these drugs at a time? This shot is the same as the pregnancy hormone hCG, which is used to predict pregnancy in over-the-counter tests. This means that if you pee on a stick within ten days, it will come back positive, even though you're not pregnant. Talk about a mind fuck, leading you to take pregnancy tests every day to see when it's out of your system so you know if it's the real deal or not. I may be crazy, but I did not do this. Do you know how expensive tests are? Waste of money. I can have patience occasionally. Then I discovered The Dollar Store!

ZOLADEX
(Gonadotropin-Releasing Hormone Analog)

The Good: Can treat endometriosis and thin the lining of the uterus before surgery.

The Bad: Hot flashes, sweating, headache, dizziness, mood changes, increased or decreased libido (well, which is it?!?), vaginal dryness/itching/discharge, breast swelling or tenderness, bone pain, diarrhea/constipation (again, which one is it?!?), sleep problems, acne, mild skin rash/itching.

The Ugly: $340 for 3.6 mg of Zoladex.

The Truth: Jesus, Mary, and Joseph! By now, you're probably thinking "Why the hell would you ever put yourself through this agony?" Simple. You want a baby. Looking back, it did take a toll on me. I'd be crying, I'd be angry, I'd be sleepy, and my feelings would be hurt. Luckily, I didn't have to take this monstrosity of a drug. But get used to these symptoms for all drugs.

I'm hopped up on hormones—happy, horny, and craving some hanky-panky. I haven't been with Noah since Chase bank. I've been sending Tinderesque messages to get his mind off babydom and make it about the exhilaration of a random hookup.

Chapter 7
Let's Get This Party Started

Today is the day I get pregnant. There are two things that I heard help conception. The first is a multivitamin called Geritol. The theory is that Geritol vitamins (yes, the ones for elderly people) are so successful at getting people pregnant that the phrase "baby in every bottle" is being thrown around. Sounds good to me! Also, I had heard that Pre-Seed personal fertility lubricant would help in conception by aiding the sperm through the cervix and into the fallopian tubes, as it mimics cervical mucus.

Side note: Not all lubricants are the same; as a matter of fact, most ingredients in lubricant kill sperm, and the thickness of lubricant makes it difficult for sperm to travel. The water content of lube can damage the sperm by causing them to absorb water. Although they can't prevent pregnancy, they are not a good choice when trying to get pregnant.

I pre-make Noah's favorite drink of Jameson and ginger ale—the one he'd ordered at the bar—and put on the Gavin DeGraw Pandora station. That's good baby-making music, right?

It's been a minute since our sexual union, and the first time was lascivious, so I'm delighted that I'll get a bit of satisfaction as well. Always love killing two birds with one stone. We talk for thirty minutes. I get tipsy and ask, "How should we do this?" I step toward him to initiate some kissing, and he steps back awkwardly.

"I'm just tired tonight. I'm gonna use my phone to get ready. Maybe you should too." I'm confused; didn't you want to sleep with me a few weeks ago? I don't understand the coldness or why it needs to be a tedious chore, but I guess I'm reading too much into this.

He stands at the bar in my kitchen and watches porn while I get my vibrator. So much for the pleasure aspect, lol.

After an eternity, a new man has risen. "So how would you want to do this?"

"However you like," I playfully state.

"Can we do it doggie?"

"Oh, so you're an ass man?" I inquire flirtatiously. He smacks my booty with his calloused hands. Thank God, this still has the potential to be enjoyable.

Once he splooges, he asks if he should stay in for a few minutes to keep from spilling out. Seems smart and practical. I knew he was intelligent. He dresses and cleans up. I put a pillow under my butt to elevate my hips, hoping gravity will help the tadpoles find their target. We awkwardly hug, and he leaves.

Just before our next scheduled "visit," Noah has worked a double shift at The Fig and requests that we postpone until the next morning. I explain that it needs to be tonight, per the timing instructions of the doctor.

I am going to up the ante: we are going to have pleasurable playtime. I have lights low, candles glowing, and The Doors Pandora station playing. Is *this* good baby-making music?

"Is there anything you want to try?" I ask.

"I liked how we did it last night."

I'm quickly disappointed. Can't a girl get a good shag without it seeming like an inconvenience? He watches porn on his phone, and I lie on my bed and play on mine, annoyed. Are there any new Snapchat filters? He slowly walks to the bed with his phone in hand and earbuds in. "Are you kidding me?" I blurt out, pissed.

45

"I want to watch for fantasy purposes." I feel icky, like a degraded piece of meat. I'm fairly quiet during coitus. I know I asked for this, but I feel humiliated right now. There is no trick and no extra attention. He finishes, goes to clean up, and gets dressed. I place the pillow under me, feeling abashed.

When he comes back from the restroom, I tell him how awkward I feel. Mind you, with the many millions of hormones I am on at this moment, it's probably the not-so-ideal situation to be bringing up. I tell him I feel like I can't touch him. He puts on his shoes. "I never mentioned you couldn't touch me."

He continues. "I started dating a friend a month ago, but don't worry about her. She's out of the country traveling." My chin trembles.

"Listen," he says, "our sex isn't meant to be romantic. We're having sex for the purpose of making a baby."

I'm embarrassed, mortified, and discouraged as my self-esteem is plummeting. "I'll stop sending flirty texts."

"You don't have to," he replies, "but I don't see our roles as being romantic."

Thanks. Got it. He leans down, kisses me on my forehead, and leaves. I guess you can't have your cake and eat it too.

My fantasies about Noah were crushed in one swift motion. I send him an apology. He tells me it wasn't a big deal and not to make it one. Everything is okay. I thought we could at least have wild, adventurous sex, not a job. After all, I want a baby, not a boyfriend.

The next day is back to normal. Leo and I are fielding phone calls from casting directors and actors. It's a lot like managing children, listening to them whine, "I overslept," "I'm running late," and "Can you get me a different audition time?" Do you know how hard it was to get you this audition? All you had to do is show up. Or do I need to be your wake-up call, too? I would be an exceptional mom.

In between calls, Leo slyly probes for information. "How's the baby making coming?" I smile and wink. He doesn't need to know I cried, lashed out, cried, apologized, and cried some more. He always knows when I'm hiding something. I hate this quality about him.

"Lisa, come on. There's something more. What are you hiding?"

I look at my phone, "Oh crap, look at the time! We're going to be late to see Roy." Roy is working as a guest star on *Scandal*. I love Kerry Washington, and I want to see where she gets her stunning coats.

Roy plays opposite Scott Foley. Man, he is *dreamy*. If this doesn't work out with Noah, maybe I can get him to batter dip the corn dog. He has great bone structure and luscious lips. Damn. Just looked him up, and the shithead is married to a model named Marika. Of course he would be.

Leo leans over. "What's wrong? What are you not telling me?"

"I looked up Scott Foley, and he is fucking married. I *am* a *little* upset."

"Lisa?"

"No, I'm just preoccupied. I'm obsessing about whether the baby dance, BD, got me pregnant."

"Glad you're now reciting acronyms." Leo is unamused.

Baby dancing is a nice, pleasant way of saying sexual intercourse, fornication, dinky-tickling, bumping uglies, makin' bacon, sinking the sausage, boinking, whoopie, and adult nap time, in case you were wondering.

Chapter 8
Symptom Spotting

WHAT IS THE TWO-WEEK WAIT?

Anyone will tell you the most difficult time between ovulation or IVF and the next expected period is the two-week wait (2WW). Every woman wants definite symptoms that show the cycle was a success and she's pregnant.

This is when women buy bulk pregnancy tests on Amazon and become pee-on-a-stick (POAS) addicts. Yes, this is an addiction. I would go to the Dollar Store and buy twenty at a time. To overcome this compulsion, I suggest not having pregnancy tests readily available. I would wake up in the morning and be like, "Hell why not try and pee?" The agony of that next five minutes always felt like an eternity. Then, when it would come back positive, I didn't know if I was really pregnant or if it was just the hCG hormone I'd been taking. Please don't become me. It's not worth the time, hassle, or money (a helpful single-girl currency-saving tip).

After fourteen days, when your next period is due, you should be able to see a positive result. Some people see it as early as nine days post-ovulation (DPO). By the time of your expected period, the trigger shot will be out of your system, and any positive will be a true positive. Typically, it takes seven to ten days, depending on how many units you injected.

DR. GOOGLE

We all are guilty of turning to Dr. Google for diagnosing every cough, pain, and even pregnancy. Who is Dr. Google? According to *Urban Dictionary*, Dr. Google is "a person medically qualified by Google's search engine to diagnose symptoms of sickness."

The best active message board for sharing and comparing symptoms during the two-week wait is on www.twoweekwait.com "Share and Compare Your Symptoms in the 2WW."

JOURNALING THE TWO-WEEK WAIT

3/13–3/14/16 4DPO–5DPO

I woke up six times to use the restroom. There was a full bladder on each occasion. I finally decided to stay awake at 2:30 a.m. Needed a nap that afternoon.

3/15/16 6DPO

Noticed more acne on my face and chest. I worked to remind myself it was caused by the 200 mg of progesterone I was taking vaginally three times daily, starting at 1DPO. I had the Ovidrel shot, which meant pregnancy hormone hCG was in my system.

I took a pregnancy test to confirm I had "tested out" (negative) of my hCG trigger and that any future positive pregnancy test result would indeed be positive.

3/16/16   7DPO

I find myself having more frequent bowel movements. This is so *not* normal.

3/17/16   8DPO

Early morning cold-like symptoms. Coughing, sore throat, hard time swallowing, frequent bowel movements. Took pregnancy test. Negative. Guess I took it too early.

I only have cramps or abdominal bloating when I lie on my stomach. Is this what pregnancy feels like?

Feeling productive and more energized than usual.

Earlier in the week, I woke up with bad headaches. That's a sign of pregnancy—or is it the progesterone? I can't keep these damn side effects straight.

3/18/16   9DPO

I woke up not feeling pregnant. Kind of losing hope for this cycle.

Had lunch with an old friend at The Grove's Cheesecake Factory. I always love going to that place. It's a well-designed outdoor shopping plaza complete with cobblestone roads and a trolley. They have a miniature version of the Bellagio water show synchronized to Rat Pack music. It's a tourist trap, but locals still enjoy it. They filmed *Extra* here, if you care. If people still watch that show. My mind completely blanked, and I ordered a Bloody Mary. During our conversation, I became overwhelmed, emotional, and lachrymose. I was gulping at air in order not to cry. There was not one reason for me to be feeling this way. I was overly teary and sensitive but not sad.

On my way home, I listened to "Piece by Piece," (Kelly Clarkson, 2015) and my eyes swelled on the verge of crying. This song is in no way relevant to me.

I watched La'Porsha Renae perform on *American Idol*, and I wept without thinking about it.

After a short bath, I was nauseated. I had to lie down. I fell asleep by 8:30 p.m. I was awakened several times by vulva itching, maybe from extra moisture. Stayed awake until 4:30 a.m.

Slept in until 10:45 a.m. This is unlike my current schedule. Tongue and back right of throat were sore again. First restroom use of the day, I had pink twinges in my cervical mucus (CM). Could this be implantation bleeding?*

*Implantation bleeding happens six to twelve days after conception, and you may mistake it for a regular period. It's light bleeding of small pink or brown spots. An early sign of pregnancy experienced by one-third of women.

Went to the editor's and had lunch with Leo. Leo and I quickly got into an argument. I became emotional—more worked up than I should be over our conversation.

Later, when talking to Leo, I became upset that he had changed plans and was no longer coming over. Then he tried to say he'd come over for a bit. I was indecisive and ultimately told him no. I was annoyed and went to sleep early. Pregnancy is certainly taking a toll on my emotional stability.

3/20/16   10DPO

I thought I was 11DPO, but upon recalculations and possible ovulation on Thursday, not Wednesday, I'll now say 10DPO. When I used the restroom, again, the toilet paper showed pink twinges in my cervical mucus.

By 5:00 p.m., I was mentally and physically wiped out, and I fell asleep for the night at 5:30 p.m. Woke up to feed the frogs and went back to bed. Had vivid dreams of being pregnant and taking a pregnancy test in my dream. Woke up at 4:30 a.m., now 11DPO, and took a pregnancy test: BFN! ☹

It's still early, I told myself. I returned to bed and woke up at 8:00 a.m. Pantyliner had light brown smudges in the middle.

After breakfast, skin-pink colored marks appeared on the toilet paper. Sharp pains dotted my lower right side with a pulling sensation.

On the set of a client's movie, felt nauseated from the smell of cigarette smoke.

3/23/16   13DPO

Took a pregnancy test—negative. I stopped taking my progesterone.

Noah and I chatted about the second cycle, potential dates, and him taking a sperm analysis test. He agreed. I didn't feel disappointed. I didn't think I'd get pregnant on the first try.

3/27/16   Started Period. FML.

To break the tension, Noah and I play Skee-Ball, ride the Ferris wheel, and share a cotton candy at the Santa Monica Pier. It's astounding how time flies with him. We can converse about nothing for hours. If I had to assign songs to the past two weeks, week one (insemination week) would be "Wicked Games" (Chris Isaak, 1990). Week two: "Almost Lover" (A Fine Frenzy, 2007).

MY IMAGINARY SYMPTOMS

These are actual real symptoms you can have. I "experienced" these during my 2WW. If you haven't realized it yet, I've included a glossary in the back of the book because I like acronyms. A lot of women, obviously including myself, have phantom symptoms because we desperately want to be pregnant.

Side note: you can trick yourself into being sick, true story.

Sneezing: Because of increased blood flow and volume, pregnant-lady noses get puffier, and pregnant women sneeze more often. FYI: Costco has a great deal on Kleenex bundles.

Crying at Dog Food Commercials: Only pregnant women cry at dog commercials, right?

Superpowers: A heightened sense of smell. I walked into a building, and swear to God, I smelled coffee. There was no coffee in sight. It must have been in another office, because there was coffee *somewhere*, I swear to you. Who smells coffee if there is no coffee? No one. That is the correct answer. No one.

Acne: Is that a pimple? I had a rash on my legs. Still don't know what the three spots on my forehead are, so I was completely convinced this was a hormone-induced breakout.

Stuffy Nose: Oh no, I have a stuffy nose this month. Hoping this is a symptom.

Blood-Flow Tits: They say when you're pregnant, the blue veins on your chest are more prominent. Prompted to do my own investigation, I legit would stand topless in front of my full-length mirror. Literally looking in the mirror, like "Hmm. Maybe. was that vein there before?"

Nipple Darkness: When you're pregnant, your nipples and areolas get darker so the baby can find its food source. True story. Once again, I found myself staring in the mirror giving myself a mammogram. How are you supposed to tell if it's darker? Am I a pepperoni? Oh wait, that's the size of the areola. How can I figure this out? I'll take a snapshot and compare. I must have a sexy photo stored somewhere.

Increased Thirst: Duh, I woke up in the middle night and drank five Gatorades—I was totes pregnant. Apparently not: I was just thirsty.

Dog's Sixth Sense: My adopted Chihuahua, Fred, kept lying on my stomach and licking inside my belly button. Does he sense something is in there? They say animals know. "They" as in, you know, *everyone*!

Ovulation Temp: I would literally run to the bathroom to take my temp. Your basal body temperature is the first temp of the day, and if it remains high, you are pregnant. I did what any normal girl would do to find out if she is pregnant: I took my temperature nine times a day, diligently.

Yawning: I yawned. Def preggo.

Hair Stops Falling Out: I wasn't shedding as much. My tumbleweeds weren't all over the floor. I must be pregnant.

Sensitivity to Certain Colors: Some women experience a distinct hate or nausea when looking at particular colors. I never liked orange—must be pregnant.

Rectal Pain: Apparently, round ligament pain can occur near the anus. This is a less common indicator you may be pregnant, but it does happen. Otherwise, probably just another hard night of partying.

Gagging When Using a Toothbrush: Some women say that as soon as they are pregnant, brushing their teeth make them gag. That has happened to everyone who brushes their tongue. Maybe don't brush so vigorously? I don't know, just a suggestion.

Sickness: My throat was sore, and I felt run down. My immune system must be weak from the baby.

Bleeding Gums: Increased blood flow makes your gums sensitive, right? I'm hoping this bleeding is from pregnancy and not gingivitis.

REAL SYMPTOMS

There are many myths out there about how pregnancy feels, and those can definitely cause women to become paranoid about symptoms.

Most natural pregnancies are not discovered until the woman misses her period (around four to six weeks). The IVF process allows women to detect if they are pregnant much sooner than a natural pregnancy; therefore, symptoms differ and are more difficult to pinpoint.

No symptom will tell you 100 percent if you are pregnant or not. The following table lists symptoms frequently reported by women during the 2WW at different stages of pregnancy. Remember: you should not overanalyze every twinge, and try to relax. Put down the pregnancy test and walk slowly away. Shut the bathroom door, sit down, and turn on the newest episode of *This Is Us*. On second thought, make that a comedy.

DURING 2WW	3–4 WEEKS	AFTER 1 MONTH
Temperature Increase	Missed Period	Lower Back Pain
Implantation Dip: Temperature Decrease	Vomiting / Nausea	Food Cravings
Spotting	Spotting	Spotting
Cramping	Cramping	Cramping
Tightness in Abdomen	Frequent Urination	Frequent Urination
Twinges in Abdomen	Breast Tenderness	Breast Tenderness
Fatigue	Fatigue	Fatigue
Headaches *	Headache	Darkened Nipples
Rash *	Stretching	Stretching
No symptoms	Emotional	Emotional
Discharge	Bloating	Constipation
Night sweats	Acne	Dizziness
		Leg Cramps

* Could be caused by the IVF medication.

Chapter 9
Back in the Saddle

That wasn't atrocious. I can do another IUI again. Dr. Nameless did a three-day ultrasound. He is making me jump through hoops. He wants to wait a cycle before we do another fertility treatment so Noah can get examined first. He also wants me to have genetic counseling—$1,100 just to say my kid could potentially have genetic disorders. What the fuck? More tests? Is this a money-making scheme I should have looked up?

Noah did not consent to this. He already seemed annoyed to be having sex with me, lol.

Rather than being disappointed, I am upbeat and positive. Maybe I will get pregnant on my own and save myself $1,000 this cycle. I decide to try the old-fashioned way.

4/2/16

I bought a First Response™ Ovulation Predictor Kit (OPK) at Ralph's.

4/4/16

Light line. Light line means ovulation is pending and you are about to ovulate.

There was no porn used today. He requested his favorite position.

I posed seductively on the bed. He grabbed my hips and adjusted my body, instructing me to lean downwards. I was vocal, and so was he. *Please, for the love of God, Lisa, don't fall for your sperm donor! It's just sex, woman! Man up!*

4/7/16

Noah missed our Wednesday and Thursday "appointments." This had me extremely worried. He said he went on a bender with his friends. He has a lot on his mind, and what we're doing has major consequences. I flipped out. I've already invested an exorbitant amount of money. Even if we move forward, we missed the best days this month. He apologized: "It won't happen again. I will make all future scheduled meetings."

4/9/16

Noah and I had another BD. Although he said it wouldn't happen again, I had a tough talk with him to make sure. This was my life now, and I needed to know he was serious, especially if he was going on benders. I didn't know what that meant for his health, which scared me even more. "This is really important to me, like, I need to know you are fully committed."

"I'm sorry. It just hit me that we're creating a child. I'm not sure I'll be able to detach from being a parent and only be a donor. I don't know how I would be able to disengage from a baby I know is mine."

"I get it's not conventional. I mean do you really see knowing this child?"

"Yeah, we're friends. Of course I'll know this child." This took me completely by surprise. I took a step back. I didn't know how to respond. I didn't know the answer. I am a great salesperson, and I didn't know how to spin this.

4/24/16   11DPO

Breakfast. I had no appetite. I love eggs, but right then they sounded disgusting. I'm hoping I'm pregnant. My friend Jennifer found out she's pregnant, and she wants an abortion. Makes me sad and upset that those who don't want a child are blessed with them and those who want them sometimes struggle.

Not sure if I'm "out of the game" this month. Noah needs to do a semen analysis, and we both need to visit Dr. Nameless at "University" hospital (obvious name change for numerous reasons) before I can continue with fertility treatments.

I needed retail therapy, and I went full force into the law of attraction. What better way than to buy baby clothes and set up a crib in your apartment? That's totally normal, right? Hey, if it doesn't work, I'll put my dogs in it for a time-out.

Noah stopped by as pieces and instructions for a crib were scattered all over my living room. He gasped at my new décor. I barked, "What? It makes me happy!" He raised his eyebrows. I pulled out an "I survived the Ice Age" onesie and baby Converses from my dresser.

Noah hesitated. "Wow, a baby will be filling that out."

"Down the road, yeah. I was feeling depressed, so I bought these for motivation. It's kinda like a vision board." Noah nodded cautiously.

"It's all good. I just have moments sometimes." Noah mustered a grin.

I explained he needs to go to the fertility clinic for some genetic testing, and he agreed without question. I didn't realize the test results would take six months due to quarantine.

Chapter 10
Let the Charades Begin

Disclaimer: Per FDA regulations, a donor (not coming from a cryobank) has to provide a sperm sample that has to be quarantined for six months. HIV takes six months to develop. Other regulations include communicable disease testing, genetic testing, and psychological evaluation at FDA-registered facilities.

This does not apply to unmarried couples in monogamous relationships. There is no way I am waiting another six months to try again.

Light bulb goes off. "We are now a couple."

In the hospital parking lot, I tell Noah there is one minor, tiny, minute, unimportant challenge we must attend to first. He glares at me with a "WTF" look.

"We need to sell that we're a couple."

Noah laughs. "Sure, whatever. Why not?"

TWENTY QUESTIONS

It's eight in the morning, and Noah is not a morning person, nor am I. Dr. Nameless watches suspiciously as Noah nervously twiddles his thumbs. I grab his hand. He awkwardly tries to hold mine.

"So, you guys met earlier this year? And you were her donor?"

Noah nods in agreement.

"We fell in love," I pipe in.

"And now you're a couple?"

"Yes." I am not missing a beat.

"Noah, why do you want a child?"

Noah pets my hair (a little overkill). "I just want her to be happy."

"Do you plan on raising this child together?"

I have Noah hanging by a string, and this damn doctor keeps asking ridiculously intrusive questions that will make him run for the hills. Does he interrogate all his couples?

"Of course," Noah says out of nowhere. I let out a huge sigh of relief. Noah clutches my leg and wide-tooth smiles at Dr. Nameless.

"What is your medical history?"

"Do you have any undescended testicles?"

"Do you have a problem ejaculating?"

"Are you able to maintain an erection?"

"Have you ever had a sexually transmitted disease?"

"What's your sexual orientation?"

"Roughly how many partners have you been with?"

"Are you willing to submit to an infectious disease panel and provide a sperm sample for analysis?"

Dr. Nameless shuts the door and asks me to undress from the waist down, as he is going to do a pelvic ultrasound. Noah's mouth falls open. He's trapped. I'm mortified. During the examination, the doctor includes Noah and shows him my follicles.

"Cool." Noah eyes the exit.

A nurse hijacks Noah. We haven't even had breakfast yet. Noah clears his throat. "Oh, now?"

Noah's sperm count was forty-five million—above average—with good motility and normal morphology. Everything looks good.

62

He's not the problem. I'm not the problem. This must be unexplained infertility. Maybe I'm not tilting my pelvis enough?

We're handed a slip with test orders and directed toward the lab. Is today ever going to end?

Noah fidgets in the lab chair as the phlebotomist pulls seven vials from the drawer. The tourniquet is tightly wrapped around his arm as he rocks in place. She attempts to insert the needle, and Noah faints. With a wet washcloth on his forehead, he comes to and blames it on needing food. We go to the cafeteria.

We're across from each other at the table. I ask, "How are you doing?"

"Mentally? I'm very far away." I don't blame him. I keep apologizing, fearing he's going to back out. Noah calms me with a soothing tone. "You have nothing to worry about."

A few days pass, and the tests are back. He is clear of any diseases. Thank God, because I had been reckless with him. The doctor said, "Let's try an IUI plus timed intercourse."

Chapter 11
Just No Saliva

IUI LOWDOWN

Intrauterine insemination (IUI) is a fertility treatment involving placing sperm inside a woman's uterus to facilitate fertilization. The goal of IUI is to increase the number of sperm reaching the fallopian tubes and, subsequently, increase the chance of fertilization.

FIRST ARTIFICIAL POLLINATION

Ten days into my cycle, after taking Clomid and having ultrasounds, I'm told to use my trigger shot to initiate ovulation. The next morning, at 7:00 a.m., Noah and I are escorted to a private room by a nurse. I'm not sure what's happening, but it soon becomes apparent: they want him to give a sperm sample. They put him in a room at seven in the morning to jerk off? But why am I in the room? The nurse hands him a cup, looks at me, and states, "Just no saliva." I'm rattled. That did not just come out of her mouth.

"I'm just going to give him some space. I'll wait outside."
We were never put in that position again, thank goodness. That was awkward. I mean, like, it was *really* awkward.

An hour later, after the sperm has been washed, I'm inseminated with Noah's gene pool.

The next day, per doctor's instructions, we have a scheduled "meeting." I stay up late the night before researching the best positions for conception, and since doggie hadn't worked, I want to try a new flavor.

I request we do missionary to increase the likelihood of it working. I mean, the Internet is never wrong, right? Noah reluctantly agrees but adds a condition: "Don't expect me to look you in the eyes or anything."

What is this, *Pretty Woman*, and you're Julia Roberts, except instead of kisses, you don't make eye contact?

I do the only normal thing to do: I shut my eyes and pretend it's Brad Pitt. I bet you *he* would look into my eyes.

MY 2WW

This two-week wait is different. I have none of my previous pregnancy symptoms, just an achy chest. Must be the jalapeños I ate last night.

Chapter 12
Am I Pregnant?

VERY FAINT SQUINTER EXPLANATION

Ten days post-ovulation, I've waited long enough. I pull one of my many pregnancy tests out of my vanity. I use first morning urine (FMU, you know, the most concentrated). I set the test on the bathroom counter and make breakfast in the kitchen. Cereal with milk.

When I approach the stick, I do a double take. Is that a second line? I quickly grab the test and hold it up to the light. Something is there! Is there color to that line, or is it an evap line? Let me take a picture.

I text a handful of girlfriends the pic and ask their opinion, hoping to get confirmation. I'm encouraged to take another test the next day. What a long twenty-four excruciating hours.

I wake up preposterously early and anxious about testing. It's Christmas morning, and Santa has brought me a present.

I open my cabinet and look at the reserve of pregnancy tests. This time I choose a good one: First Response! Within two minutes, a second pink line appears, not nearly as dark as the control line, but it's certainly there.

Elated, I call the doctor's office, and the nurse books a blood test: a quantitative hCG test (beta hCG is ordered).

POAS PREGNANCY TEST SENSITIVITY

When looking for a pregnancy test, especially when you plan to test early, you want to choose an extra-sensitive one. By sensitive, I mean it detects pregnancy with lower levels of hCG: pregnancy from 10–50 mIU. You will get a positive pregnancy sooner with the 10 vs. the 50.

Baby Test (Dollar Store)	20 mIU
Clearblue Easy	25 mIU
CVS (cartridge)	25 mIU
CVS (stick test)	25 mIU
e.p.t.	25 mIU
Equate (Wal*Mart)	25 mIU
Equate (Wal*Mart)	25 mIU
First Response Early Result	15–25 or 6.3 mIU
New Choice (Dollar Tree)	20 mIU
Rite-Aid	25 mIU
Target	25 mIU
Walgreens	25 mIU
Clearblue Easy Digital (U.S.)	50 mIU
Dollar General Store	50 mIU
e.p.t. 1Step*	40 mIU
e.p.t. Certainty digital	50 mIU
Family Dollar	50 mIU
Rite-Aid	50 mIU
Target	50 mIU
Walgreens	50 mIU

WHAT IS A BETA TEST?

There are two common types of hCG tests. A qualitative hCG test detects if hCG is present in the blood. A quantitative hCG test, often called a beta test, measures the amount of hCG actually present in the blood.

It doesn't matter what your starting number is as long as the number continues to double every forty-eight hours.

BLOOD TEST LOW

Four hours later, I receive a call from the nurse letting me know that, indeed, I am technically pregnant, but the beta number is relatively low, measuring in at twelve.

I ask if she's ever witnessed a healthy pregnancy continue with a low starting number. Her blasé response: "It can happen, but rarely." Using anger to feed my strength, I stay confident. She orders another blood test for forty-eight hours later.

BETA NUMBER RANGE

hCG levels in weeks from the last normal menstrual period:

3 weeks LMP	5 – 50 mIU/ml
4 weeks LMP	5 – 426 mIU/ml
5 weeks LMP	18 – 7,340 mIU/ml
6 weeks LMP	1,080 – 56,500 mIU/ml
7-8 weeks LMP	7, 650 – 229,000 mIU/ml

*LMP means last menstrual period. It also shows how many weeks pregnant you are.

During that forty-eight hours, I relish the thought that I am, quote, unquote, "pregnant." It must have been the missionary position.

The results for the second blood test come back quicker. Rather than doubling, it has decreased to eight. This confirms that I had a chemical pregnancy.

WHAT IS A CHEMICAL PREGNANCY?

A chemical pregnancy is actually a very early miscarriage, and it happens before anything can be seen on an ultrasound scan, usually around the fifth week of pregnancy. It means a sperm has fertilized your egg, but later on, the egg fails to survive.

Why is this so difficult? It has been six months. I should be pregnant by now. I have a doctor helping me. I'm injecting myself and having sex more often than an NBA All-Star. I don't get it. Little do I know there is a lot more to learn.

Chapter 13
This Isn't Working

It's now September, and we've performed two more IUI cycles and timed intercourse, with no luck. Doctors recommend doing six IUI cycles before moving on. I've done three. Between treatment, medication, and donor sperm, I'm spending $2,100 per cycle.

In my mind, I had gotten pregnant the first cycle. Am I going to have to wait another six cycles for it to work again? The percentage doesn't go up every time you do it; it's an average. If you do it six times, you're likely to get pregnant once.

I'm on *The Lovers* film set, shooting at a house in Santa Clarita. This part of LA feels more Midwestern. They even have an Applebee's! Bring on happy hour prices! There's more camaraderie, and people put their families before their careers.

The home is owned by a family of five with three boys, the youngest being two and a half. The mother's name is Kimberly. She's in her early forties, beautiful, tall, with long, dark hair. She is incredibly sweet, and you want to hug her instantly. She teaches psychiatry at a local college, and she speaks with sass and truth.

After a week of filming, we develop a friendship. I fall in love with her two-year-old. He is a snuggle bug. One day when she's holding him, Kimberly inquires about my desire for children. Oh, boy, she doesn't know what can of worms she's opening!

I tell her about my failed IUI, TIs, and medicated cycles. I'm close to giving up. My doctor is cold and unresponsive. He doesn't seem to truly care whether or not I become a mom. She sympathizes, and I think, *You have no idea.* Little do I know she is the guru of fertility treatments. Her first son was a Clomid and timed intercourse baby. Her second son was an IUI baby, and her third was an IVF miracle.

She comforts me. "It will come when the time is right, and maybe you needed to meet me to realize it is time to change doctors."

She insists her doctor is the most kind, compassionate, and caring man she's ever met. She relentlessly encourages me to meet him, even stating she will go with me for the first consultation.

I contemplate her suggestion, knowing I don't like my doctor's bedside manner. I Google her doctor's information and make an appointment.

Chapter 14
The Fertility Truth

It's 8:30 a.m. on a Thursday. Kimberly greets me in the lobby of her former doctor—whom we will be calling Dr. Know-it-all—toting her youngest son, Jonah. Doctors love it when you bring in the baby they created. This is his first time meeting Jonah. He is delighted to see Jonah. He coos over him and reminisces with Kimberly. Not a bad first impression.

At Dr. Know-it-all's desk, pictures of his own children are displayed with pride. I hand him my welcome packet and my fertility medical records from "University" hospital. He literally examines each page of every test and reads thoroughly. I eagerly wait. "Have you ever had injectables?"

This perplexes me. I've only read about those medications. Dr. Know-it-all seems surprised, and I'm not sure why. After he completes his review, he closes my file. He takes a moment, trying to figure out the right words to tell me what he's found.

"Lisa, umm, I do see a few problems with your charts." My heart sinks. He mentions my anti-Müllerian hormone (AMH) and how it is unusually low.

"Well isn't that good? I don't have malaria."

"No, Lisa, that gives us an insight into your ovarian reserve. In my opinion, you have premature ovarian failure." I'm confused. Why am I just finding this out now, when the other doctor had this test? The bad news keeps rolling. "Your follicle-stimulating hormone is too high."

"Doesn't that mean it was going to stimulate my follicles more?"

Again, "No, it actually means your eggs are absolute shit." He might have not said "shit," but my ears hear differently. You know how bad news comes in threes? "And lastly, your right fallopian tube is blocked, reducing your chances of pregnancy by 50 percent."

I recap in my head. *So basically, I don't have many eggs, the ones I have are trash, and I can only get pregnant from my left ovary?*

"Your only option to get pregnant is IVF. I'm surprised you've never heard this before. You won't get pregnant from an IUI."

"I'm confused. Why was I doing IUIs when 50 percent of the time I only had follicles on my right side?"

Dr. Know-it-all is puzzled, "With your right fallopian tube being closed, that never would have worked." He adds that I should try to lose 10 percent of my weight, as that will increase conception rates. I think he's crazy until, upon further research, I discover that many clinics have cutoffs for BMI.

We do a vaginal ultrasound to check my follicles. I have an antral follicle (AFC) of six, which means how many eggs are beginning. We go back to his office, and he says to me, "Even with IVF, you would probably only get nine or ten eggs at retrieval." That sounds like a lot until he explains that some women get more than thirty! He stresses again that not only is IVF my only option, I'm also on borrowed time. At any point, my body could stop responding, and we will not get eggs.

I regret the six months I've wasted with Dr. Nameless at "University" hospital, not to mention the money spent and the emotional roller coaster.

Here is a list of tests and what you should ask your doctor, since, apparently, they aren't always forthcoming with the results. I thought everything was fine. Isn't it the doctor's responsibility to tell you if a test comes up abnormal? I guess not. Please don't be as naïve as I was, and be your own advocate.

BATTERY OF FERTILITY TESTING

DHEA-Sulfate: DHEA is a circulating steroid in humans produced in the adrenal glands. Later on, we will talk about using DHEA as a supplement. This checks your levels.

17-Alfa-OH Progesterone: High levels of this progesterone can cause a glandular disorder resulting in the adrenal glands being unable to create sufficient cortisol, and it may increase the production of male sex hormones, called androgens.

Testosterone Total Free: Measures the amount of testosterone in your body.

Progesterone: Progesterone levels are checked to confirm ovulation.

VZV AB Immune Status: VZV stands for varicella zoster virus, better known as herpes, chicken pox, or shingles.

Rubella AB Immune Status: Checks to make sure you have the rubella antibody and makes sure you are immune to it.

Measles AB Immune Status: Checks to make sure you have the measles antibody and makes sure you are immune to it.

HTLV I/II AB SCRN with Confirm: You will shit when you find out what it is. HTLV is a family of viruses that are a group of human retroviruses known to cause a type of cancer called adult T-Cell leukemia/lymphoma and a demyelinating disease called HTLV-1 associated with myelopathy/tropical spastic paraparesis. In my layman's opinion, this could be the next HIV.

Prolactin: To check the levels of prolactin, a protein best known for its role in enabling mammals, usually females, to produce milk.

Anti-Müllerian Hormone ASSESSR: AMH is a substance produced by granulosa cells in ovarian follicles. Remember: low means not good.

Follicle-Stimulating Hormone: A hormone secreted by the anterior pituitary gland promoting the formation of ova or sperm. The higher your FSH, the closer you are to menopause. It also shows the quality of the egg. I thought since the number was higher it would help the eggs, but it meant my eggs were shit. Remember: high means no bueno.

Estradiol: It measures the amount of estrogen in your body.

Chlamydia Trachomatis PCR: Just your basic chlamydia test.

HPVDNA: It is done to check for a high-risk HPV infection in women.

Neisseria Gonorrhoeae PCR: Again, just basically checking for your run-of-the-mill STD (i.e., putting your past into question).

Calcium for PTH: It's checking for your parathyroid function. This controls bone and blood calcium.

PTH, Intact: Another parathyroid test.

PCH, Intact and Calcium: This is used in making the diagnosis of primary and secondary hyperparathyroidism.

Vitamin D 25 Hydroxy: Checks for vitamin D deficiency.

Free T3: This is testing your actual thyroid and function.

Free T4: This, also, tests thyroid function.

TSH: Thyroid-stimulating hormone. It is necessary to have your thyroid levels balanced in order to get pregnant.

Comprehensive Metabolic Panel: Checks your sugar, electrolytes, fluid balance, kidney function, liver function, and a bunch of other miscellaneous factors. The testing is usually done at general practitioner appointments.

N-Telopeptide, Urine: It is used to assess bone health in women.

Alkaline Phosphatase: This test measures the amount of alkaline phosphate enzyme in your blood stream. High levels of ALP can indicate liver disease or bone disorders.

Bilirubin Total: It detects an increase of bilirubin in the blood. It may be used to help determine the cause of jaundice and/or help diagnose conditions such as liver disease, hemolytic anemia, and blockage of the bile ducts.

ALT: Checks for liver damage.

AST: Another indicator of liver damage or injury from different types of diseases.

HSG: A hysterosalpingogram (HSG) is a special kind of X-ray used to evaluate female fertility. It involves placing an iodine-based dye through the cervix and taking X-rays. These X-rays help evaluate the shape of the uterus and whether the fallopian tubes are blocked. You should be warned that this will hurt *so fucking bad*. It makes your uterus contract. Is this what labor feels like? Oh, and also prepare for blood afterwards. Please, please, for the love of God, ask about these results. Don't assume everything is okay. Trust me, Dr. Nameless cost me thousands upon thousands of dollars in wasted treatments because he didn't tell me my fallopian tube was blocked.

FEMALE FERTILITY TESTING PROCESS

This is what to expect from your first consultation with a reproductive endocrinologist.

During this appointment, your medical history and lifestyle will be discussed in depth—topics such as birth control use, menstrual and pregnancy history, current and past sexual practices, medications used, and surgical history. Other health issues, what your lifestyle is like, and your work/living environment will be discussed.

A thorough physical exam will be done. Your thyroid, breasts, and hair growth will be looked at. Plus, don't forget a pelvic exam and a pap smear.

You will track your ovulation through fertility-awareness apps or an at-home fertility monitor. Usually, one of the first questions regarding female fertility is whether you are ovulating or not.

Along with the above tests, here are other tests you will also encounter.

Ovulation Testing: Confirm if ovulation is occurring by looking through your temperature charts and using ovulation predictor kits, blood tests, and ultrasound.

Ovarian Function Tests: Tests to see how the hormones are functioning and working during your ovulation cycle. Tests include the day 3 FSH, day 3 estradiol (measuring estrogen), ultrasound (to confirm ovulation occurred), and blood tests to determine the levels of inhibin B. Inhibin B is a hormone produced by certain cells in the ovarian follicles directly reflecting the number of follicles in the ovary.

Luteal Phase testing: Testing will evaluate progesterone levels, more extensive hormone testing, and possibly an endometrial biopsy.

Endometrial Biopsy: A procedure involving scraping a small amount of tissue from the endometrium just prior to menstruation.

This procedure is performed to determine if the lining is thick enough for a fertilized egg to implant and grow. It is important to confirm you are not pregnant before this test is performed.

Hormone Tests: Ones on the previous page, plus luteinizing hormone and androstenedione.

Cervical Mucus Tests: A postcoital test (PCT) determines if the sperm is able to penetrate and survive in the cervical mucus. It also involves a bacterial screening.

Ultrasound Tests: Used to assess the thickness of the lining of the uterus (endometrium), to monitor follicle development, and to check the condition of the uterus and ovaries. An ultrasound may be conducted two to three days later to confirm an egg has been released.

Hysteroscopy: This procedure may be used if the HSG indicates the possible presence of abnormalities. The hysteroscope is inserted through the cervix into the uterus, which allows your fertility specialist to see any abnormalities, growths, or scarring in the uterus. The hysteroscope allows the physician to take pictures and can be used for future reference.

Laparoscopy: A procedure done under general anesthesia and involves the use of a narrow fiber optic telescope. The laparoscope is inserted into a woman's abdomen to provide a view of the uterus, fallopian tubes, and ovaries. If any abnormalities such as endometriosis, scar tissue, or other adhesions are found, they can be removed by a laser. It is important to confirm you are not pregnant before this test is performed.

After the appointment, I go home with a torrential downpour running down my face. I can't believe how much I didn't know about my own fertility. Turns out I *am* the problem.

I call Leo the instant I get home. Right when I hear his soothing voice, I burst into waterworks. Seeking comfort in his words, "Everything will work out. You know I'm always here for you, baby," I crawl into bed. Hopefully, I'll wake up and this is all a bad dream.

Chapter 15
18K in Three Days

Leo is at my door with flowers and bagels in hand. Now that I've processed the news, I've become determined to attempt IVF. My cycle is in three days. I desperately want to prep for IVF this upcoming cycle, as I know with every cycle that passes, my chances of pregnancy dwindle.

Here comes the sticker shock. I am *not* prepared for how much IVF actually costs. With this doctor, the cycle is *$11,000*, preimplantation genetic screening (PGS) testing is *$3,500* for eight embryos (see Chapter 18 for explanation), and medication is between *$4,000* and *$6,000*. I'm looking at a minimum of $18,000 for *one* IVF cycle.

How in the world am I going to get $18,000 in three days? I don't have a choice. I don't have enough time to apply for a grant. If you want a list of available grants for IVF, visit Fertility Authority (fertilityauthority.com). Also, check with your insurance company, as some offer full or partial fertility coverage.

Fun fact: Starbucks covers IVF and other fertility treatments for its employees, even part-time ones. I've read many stories of women getting second jobs at Starbucks just for the fertility coverage. For more information, visit the Facebook page "Starbucks IVF Mommas." If only I had heard of this sooner.

I don't have $18K in my bank account, and my credit is not strong enough to get approved by a fertility finance company. (Inquire at your fertility clinic as to which fertility finance companies they work with, and expect to pay a higher interest rate. My loan has a set amount of interest, whether I pay it off early or follow the payment schedule of the loan.)

The nurses told me about Compassionate Care, where income-qualified patients can receive a discount code for certain fertility medications (fertilitylifelines.com). Another similar company is called First Steps (fertilitybydesign.com). Definitely look into them before purchasing any medication.

The hardest predicament you'll ever have is to ask your family for money. I've always been independent and self-sufficient, and I've prided myself on being financially responsible—sometimes. I have to swallow my pride, as I have no other choice.

My sister has been my source of support from the beginning and knows how desperately I want to be a mom. She is my sounding board, my rock. It takes a few phone calls, and yes, in one day, I call her seventeen times. She lets me know she doesn't have the cash but she has the credit. My internal struggle is hoping she just has the money and I don't have to worry. My sister has everything: a jewelry store, jet skis, boats, and a house on nine acres with a barn. I think she has the money lying around. Now that I know it's going on credit, what if something happens and I can't pay it? But what if I miss this cycle and this is the only opportunity I have to get pregnant? I already know that adoption is not an option.

My inner monologue wrestles with guilt. *Am I being selfish because I want a baby more than anything? I wish she had boosted a "no problem." I now feel pressure for this to work. I told her this was my whole life. Have I become obsessive? My primal instinct is kicking in. I am a woman. My soul purpose is to be able to bear children.* According to the book *The Female Brain*, biology can hijack the circuits in our brain in spite of our best intentions, especially if we have been trying for a while. It's called mommy brain.

My sister hesitantly acquiesces and is approved for a fertility loan. The money is wired straight to the doctor's office.

The doctors take their portion and cut me a check for the balance so I can pay the pharmacy directly for the fertility drugs.

Noah comes over and sees how I am after the devastating news. He pulls out his guitar and serenades me with a rendition of "Patience" (Guns N' Roses, 1988). Is he singing about me or the process? Either way, I'm starting to get the feels, and I have no hormone medicine to blame. Can we practice a baby dance now? Just kidding, but really not even a little bit.

What Noah is thinking: *Said woman take it slow, and it'll work itself out fine. All we need is just a little patience.*

What Lisa hears: "Girl, I think about you every day now. There's no doubt you're in my heart. We'll come together."

Revived after Noah's regaling performance, I am ready to do anything and everything I need to do to get pregnant, including gulping horse pills and consuming all the holistic grossness.

Chapter 16
Vitamins up the Hoo-Ha

I HOPE YOU LIKE TO SWALLOW

Countless women idolize the book *It Starts with an Egg: How the Science of Egg Quality Can Help You Get Pregnant Naturally, Prevent Miscarriage, and Improve Your Odds in IVF* by Rebecca Fett. Dr. Know-it-all hands me a list of vitamins and supplements he recommends. You have to take the vitamins for at least three months to improve egg quality. I end up taking these gargantuan pellets for over a year.

ANTIOXIDANTS
Antioxidants protects cells from free radicals. All of the organs, fluids, and players in the reproductive system are made up of cells, which need protecting. Healthy cells = healthy fertility.

Coenzyme Q10: Occurs naturally in our body. It helps production of adenosine triphosphate (ATP) molecules, which act as the energy currency of our cells. Aging egg cells have defective energy production, so supplementing CoQ10 is beneficial for women of advanced maternal age. There are many claims about CoQ10, including aneuploidy (we will explain aneuploidy in Chapter 18) prevention, increased egg yield, better egg quality, and so on. Foods: Liver, kidney, heart, beef, sardines, mackerel, spinach, broccoli, cauliflower, peanuts, and soybeans.

R-Alpha Lipoic Acid: In high-risk pregnancies, lipoic acid can speed up the return to normal pregnancy conditions and improve the conditions of both the mother and the fetus. Additionally, a smaller number of miscarriages were recorded with lipoic acid supplementation. Lipoic acid reduced cervical inflammation after a preterm labor episode. Foods: Spinach, broccoli, tomato, kidney, liver, heart.

Pycnogenol: A strong antioxidant derived from the bark of the pine tree. It helps the quality of sperm and increases sperm count. Since it is assumed free radicals cause damage to eggs, this antioxidant supplement is important among women undergoing IVF. Foods: Grapes, blueberries, cherries, plums, leaves of the hazelnut tree, barks of the lemon tree and the Landis pine tree. (These are very small and insignificant amounts, unfortunately.)

Resveratrol: May have a role in preserving fertility, protecting immature egg cells, and potentially extending the fertile years. Foods: Blueberries, mulberries, and skins of red grapes.

Melatonin: Eggs, like all cells in the human body, are exposed to free radicals that can cause DNA damage. Melatonin actually acts as an antioxidant in the ovaries, removing free radicals and preventing cellular damage. The suggested dose for women who are undergoing IVF is 3 mg/day. This is a major issue on IVF boards. You should not take too much, but if you don't take enough, it's not effective. Goldilocks really did have a dilemma on her hands. Foods: Tart cherries, corn, asparagus, tomatoes, pomegranates, olives, grapes, broccoli, cucumbers, rice, barley, rolled oats, walnuts, peanuts, sunflower seeds, mustard seeds, flaxseed.

Vitamin C: High levels of ascorbic acid present in the ovaries may be responsible for collagen synthesis, which is required for follicle and corpus luteum growth as well as repair of the ovary post-ovulation. Problems with this function may contribute to the development of ovarian cysts.

Ascorbic acid has also been shown to greatly impact the integrity of the follicle membrane and wall. Other research shows a correlation between serum ascorbic acid levels and follicular fluid levels in women undergoing IVF at the time of oocyte recovery. Adequate intake of vitamin C is essential for maintaining a healthy menstrual cycle and maintaining or improving egg health. Foods: Acerola cherries, guava, mustard greens, parsley, persimmons, papayas, bell peppers, broccoli, brussels sprouts, strawberries, oranges, kiwifruits, cauliflower, kale, elderberries, spinach, red cabbage, potatoes, tomatoes, and citrus fruits.

Vitamin E: Helps increase the thickness of the wall of the uterus. Helps stimulate egg cell production in women with unexplained infertility. Vitamin E increases the thickness in the uteruses of the patients. Foods: Wheat germ oil, sunflower seeds, almonds, hazelnuts, spinach, avocados, turnip greens, butternut squash, pine nuts, palm oil, peanuts, olive oil, mangos, sweet potatoes, tomatoes.

Selenium: Helps to protect the eggs and sperm from free radicals. Selenium is also necessary for the creation of sperm. In studies, men with low sperm counts have also been found to have low levels of selenium. Foods: Brazil nuts, yellowfin tuna, halibut, sardines, grass-fed beef, turkey (boneless), beef liver, chicken, eggs, spinach.

Zinc: In women, zinc works with more than three hundred different enzymes in the body to keep things working well. Without it, your cells can not divide properly; your estrogen and progesterone levels can get out of balance, and your reproductive system may not be fully functioning. Low levels of zinc have been linked to miscarriage in the early stages of a pregnancy. Foods: Lamb, pumpkin seeds, grass-fed beef, chickpeas, cocoa powder, cashews, kefir or yogurt, mushrooms, spinach, chicken.

INSULIN SENSITIZERS

Women with polycystic ovarian disease (PCOD) have insulin resistance. Excess insulin in the body can disrupt hormonal balance, leading to lack of periods. Insulin sensitizers like metformin are proven effective in inducing ovulation and therefore help women with PCOD to get pregnant. They also improve egg quality in normal women.

Myo-Inositol: Myo-inositol prevents folate-resistant neural tube defects (NTD), which are defects in the brain, spine, or spinal cord. Women who had children with NTD even after consuming enough folates could try a myo-inositol supplement too. It is a vitamin B-complex supplement. Foods: Cantaloupe, citrus fruits (other than lemons), oats, and bran.

Cinnamon Extract: Greatly reduces insulin resistance in women with PCOS.

Apple Cider Vinegar: Helps maintain an alkaline pH in both your saliva and your vaginal environment to facilitate conception. In addition, it helps treat candida, which may lead to infertility.

PCOD MIMETIC

While PCOD women have a lot of antral follicles in their ovaries, not all women have a high antral count.

DHEA: Helps women with low antral follicle counts to produce more eggs. It is also thought DHEA helps reduce chromosomal abnormalities, resulting in better egg and embryo quality and a reduction in miscarriage. Foods: Ghee, raw butter, cod liver oil, coconut oil, red palm oil, flaxseed oil, evening primrose oil, pumpkin seeds, and olive oil.

Not-so-fun fact: according to Columbia University's Health Services, DHEA may cause women to grow excess facial hair when taken in excessive doses (more than 100 mg per day), and it may deepen their voices.

VITAMINS, MINERALS, AND AMINO ACIDS

Necessary for the optimal functioning of the body, so it is necessary for the reproductive system as well.

Prenatal Vitamins: Help with any nutritional gaps in diet. Crucial for maintaining healthy fertility.

Vitamin D: Shown to increase AMH level, the hormone is a marker for ovarian reserve. Foods: Spinach, kale, okra, collards, soybeans, white beans, sardines, salmon, perch, rainbow trout, tuna, mackerel, orange juice, soy milk, beef liver, cheese, egg yolks.

Vitamin B-Complex: Helps regulate menstrual cycles, produce less painful periods, and improve egg quality. Foods: Liver, legumes, dried beans, fresh orange juice, rice, fish, red meat, eggs, poultry, milk, milk products, cheese, soy products.

Folic Acid: Every woman trying to conceive should take folic acid. It is proven to prevent neural tube defects in the developing fetus. Folic acid prevents 70 percent of neural tube defects. Take 400 mg of folic acid daily for at least three months prior to starting your IVF treatment.

Women with a mutation in their methylenetetrahydrofolate gene (MTFHR)—yes, that is one word—need 500 mg of folic acid daily in order to protect their fetus against neural tube defects. MTFHR gene mutation can inhibit an important metabolic process called methylation. This process converts folate and folic acid into an active form a body can use. Women who have MTFHR gene mutation have to take more. Foods: Dark leafy greens, asparagus, broccoli, papayas, oranges, grapefruits, strawberries, raspberries, beans, peas, lentils, avocadoes, okra, brussels sprouts, sunflower seeds, peanuts, flaxseeds, almonds, cauliflower, beets, corn, celery, carrots, squash.

Biotin: Some women might experience biotin deficiency while taking fertility drugs, so it is recommended to take biotin to restore it. Hair loss and brittle nails aren't the best. Foods: Beef liver, eggs, salmon, sunflower seeds, sweet potatoes, almonds, tuna, spinach, broccoli, cheddar cheese, milk, plain yogurt, oatmeal, bananas.

Calcium: Vital ingredient in the process of triggering growth in embryos. The more calcium in the surrounding fluid, the better. Foods: Raw milk, yogurt, figs, spinach, salmon, almond butter, sesame seeds, turnip greens, bok choy, kale, blackstrap molasses, and white beans.

L-Arginine/L-Ornithine/L-Lysine: Amino acids often taken by couples facing fertility issues. The body is able to make L-arginine, though dietary intake is important for ensuring you have enough of this amino acid. Good dietary sources include nuts, lentils, kidney beans, and fresh soybeans. It is used to increase blood circulation to the uterus, ovaries, and genitals. Can increase sperm production in men. Improves production of cervical mucus and supports a healthy libido. I'm in! Foods: Turkey, pork loin, chicken, pumpkin seeds, soybeans, peanuts, spirulina, dairy, chickpeas, lentils, beans, legumes, fish, quinoa, pistachios.

BLOOD THINNERS

An anticoagulant like a low-dose aspirin improves blood circulation to the uterus and can help in the development of a good endometrial lining. By thinning the blood, they are thought to help embryo implantation, too.

ESSENTIAL FATTY ACIDS

Fatty acids are important for the viability, maturity, and functional characteristics of sperm. Can decrease FSH levels in women, which we talked about earlier in the book. Can help improve egg quality, and could prolong reproductive function into an advanced age. Positively affects the neurodevelopment of the fetus.

Omega 3: Helps fertility by regulating hormones in the body, increasing cervical mucus, promoting ovulation, and overall improving the quality of the uterus by increasing the blood flow to the reproductive organs. Foods: Firm tofu, spinach, fontina cheese, navy beans, grass-fed beef, anchovies, mustard seeds, walnuts, winter squash, eggs, purslane, flaxseed oil, wild rice, chia seeds, red lentils, and fish.

Evening Primrose Oil: May increase the quality of cervical mucus, making it a more fertile medium for sperm.

Note: Evening primrose oil should only be taken from menstruation to ovulation, as EPO may cause uterine contractions. The dosage taken should be 1500 mg to 3000 mg per day.

OTHER MISCELLANEOUS SUBSTANCES

These substances reduce stress, improve mental health, act as a tonic, flush out toxins, boost immunity, and improve the general well-being of the body and our reproductive system!

Vitex: Helps with a range of issues such as PMS, low progesterone, lack of ovulation, irregular menstrual cycles, and lack of a menstrual cycle. For PMS, take 400 mg daily before breakfast. For endometriosis, take 400 mg twice daily.

Royal Jelly: Contains royalactin, a protein found to give the queen bee its phenomenal reproductive capacity. Worker bees live an average of thirty days; the queen bee lives upwards of six years. How can she live off this exclusively? It tastes like shit.

Wheat Grass: An excellent source of nutritional antioxidants, including vitamin C, vitamin E, chlorophyll, and trace amounts of beta-carotene and selenium.

Nettle Leaf and Red Raspberry Leaf Tea: Help to tone the muscles of the pelvic region, including the uterus. This is a wonderful action for improving uterine health where uterine weakness is present. When used in preparation for pregnancy, these may help prevent miscarriage due to uterine weakness. They are also a great source of calcium, as many fertility specialists want you to eliminate dairy from your diet. Even though these are amazing herbs, I read that they should not be taken during pregnancy. I know, you can't always believe what you read on the Internet—guilty.

Most doctors don't want you taking herbs, as some are extremely powerful and potent. Please check.

Probiotics: Help with infections, balance pH levels, and improve IVF outcomes and fertility through management of pathogenic bacterial infections. Use of probiotics minimizes pregnancy complications, reduces systemic inflammation, and decreases preterm births. Foods: Kefir, sauerkraut, kimchi, kombucha, coconut kefir, natto, kvass, apple cider vinegar, brine-cured olives, tempeh, miso.

IVF PREPARATION KITS

These kits are costlier and don't always include the proper supplements. Another helpful single-girl tip: buy the vitamins yourself and separate them.

SUPPLEMENTS FOR SPERM COUNT AND MOTILITY

Zinc; vitamins C, E, and B-12; L-arginine; L-carnitine; maca; ginseng; folic acid; horny goat weed. (This last herb is known to have a powerful effect on the sexual desire of both men and women. It is believed to raise testosterone levels as well as treat erectile dysfunction in men, and increases in sperm production and semen are also benefits you can get from this powerful aphrodisiac. This can be purchased on Amazon, at GNC, or from your local drugstore. You are welcome.)

Disclaimer: Please research and consult your doctor before taking any of these supplements. Many could have side effects if taken in excess.

Chapter 17
All on a Tank of Gas

My client, Katelin, a broadcast journalism student at Cal State LA, asks me if she can do a documentary on IVF for her class final. She begins documenting the process from day one of the cycle, starting with stimulation.

(PAPER)WORK, (PAPER)WORK, (PAPER)WORK

How excited are you going to be, filling out forty-four pages of paperwork? You better learn how to initial. Work on that celebrity autograph.

They will ask questions you never even thought of. My favorite question:

Upon death, what do you want to have happen with your future children? (Embryos)
* ❖ Dispose of them.
* ❖ Donate to an infertile couple/individual.
* ❖ Donate for research purposes.

❖ Make available to a designated person. I'm sure Leo would want them.

❖ Other disposition that is clearly stated. For those of you who want to make your embryos into jewelry. True fact: people are putting their embryos into necklaces. I'm not into fashion, but I'm gonna go with that is not "in."

STEM CYCLE LOWDOWN

The period of time before your LH surge/ovulation in which the doctor prescribes medication to stimulate the ovaries, resulting in high quantity and stronger follicles.

CAN YOU FOLLOW INSTRUCTIONS?

New doctor. Same tests. Noah and I are irritated we have to do this over, but I guess I get it. I don't really, though. They have our test results from the other doctor. I don't get it. Do you get it? Yeah, no? Me neither.

I have a meeting with the nurse, who goes over my IVF medication protocol. She also shows me how to administer each injection. Certain medicines require mixing and measuring—fun! Thank goodness she's printed out instruction sheets. It's too much information to retain. Dr. Know-it-all decides on an antagonist protocol for my situation.

There are two different medication protocols for IVF stimulation: the agonist and antagonist. Please consult your doctor to decide which is best suited to your condition.

The antagonist medications I used were birth control, Clomid, Menopur, Gonal-F, Cetrotide, and Ovidrel.

Many online pharmacies ship nationwide. Since LA is the epicenter, many of these companies are based locally. One pharmacy is MDR. This is a "fertility" pharm, and *everything* is pregnancy related. I mean, they have pregnancy tests, vitamins, cocoa butter for stretch marks, and Preggie Pops for morning sickness. If you need it, they have it. No matter what shelf you look on, it's all fertility related.

At the counter, welcomed by a friendly face and a $4,200 bill, I grudgingly hand over my debit card, expecting a bag full of medicine. The pharmacist comes around the corner holding a cooler—not a kid's lunch pail cooler, a "we are going to the beach" cooler. *Massive.* I didn't realize most of this medication requires dry ice. While I'm carrying the Styrofoam boat, the damn handle breaks. I crack up laughing. What else do you do in this situation? Laughter is the best medicine. Get it? Great pun, Lisa, great pun!

Once home, I organize the medicine into a door-hanging caddy that stretches to the floor. It has my needles, swabs, alcohol wipes, the nonrefrigerated medicine, and my vitamins. I empty the veggie drawer in the fridge and stack the vials by category.

It's the first night, and I've already forgotten what the nurse said. Each medication has different instructions, such as: take a syringe with a q-tab, draw the fluid out of one vial, insert that fluid into a vial of powder, gently roll the vial because it can't be shaken, apply a large needle to take out the concoction, switch it to a smaller-gauge needle, take an alcohol swab, and insert the needle in the appropriate area. Now tell me the first thing I said. Don't cheat. I have to do this with multiple medications for ten nights. After three days, I return to the fertility clinic to check my follicles and hormone levels.

I am down to my last $20 until my next check. This normally wouldn't be a problem, but this clinic is in Thousand Oaks. That is far! It's in a whole other county! Trust me, without traffic, this is going to take me an hour. How long will $20 of gas last? I am about to find out, haha. Oh, shit, what am I doing? I am doing a $20,000 procedure, and I have $20 to my name. I mean, sounds logical.

NOT READY TO THROW IN THE TOWEL

Katelin films my ultrasound today. Expecting to have super-sized follicles on steroids, I am told it is quite the opposite. My body isn't responding to the meds. Dr. Know-it-all decides to give it a few more days.

Still on the same tank of gas, Katelin and I voyage back two days later. They do bloodwork, testing my estrogen and progesterone. They do another ultrasound to see if my follicles have begun to grow. Unfortunately, one is much larger than the others, which means one follicle is absorbing most of the medicine (this is called a dominant follicle). You want all of the follicles to grow at the same rate. When they are all mature, you can trigger their release. With a lead follicle, if the others don't catch up, they have to cancel the cycle. Dr. Know-it-all agrees to wait a few more days to see how the other follicles grow, but he isn't optimistic. He actually pats my hand. "I really want this to happen for you. We are going to try."

I am devastated. It's the first time I have a breakdown. Genuinely, I'm a sobbing, blubbery mess. Uncertainty washes over me, parading its ugly head. "It isn't going to work, Lisa. You aren't meant to be a mom." Assuming worst-case scenarios, where is Tony Robbins when you need a pep talk? Positive affirmations, positive affirmations. *My uterus loves me. My follicles are all maturing at the same rate. I have beautiful, glistening, ripe eggs, ready to be fertilized.*

This is my only shot. I don't know if the doctor will give me a refund. I've already opened the medicine, so I'm out of pocket for that. If this doesn't work, I'm done. I've played all my cards. What does a panic attack feel like?

Katelin decides this is the perfect moment to document. I'm bawling. My emotions deserve an Oscar. I can tell she's thrilled with the footage.

On Sunday, Dr. Know-it-all isn't on call, so I have another doctor do my ultrasound, and since he isn't my doctor, he won't tell me what he saw. He'll give the information to Dr. Know-it-all and let him decide what to do. Great. I get to wait again? I'm riddled with anxiety. Does time feel like it's slowing down? *Hey Lisa, I have an idea. Why don't we replay every facial expression that doctor made while he was looking at your uterus. Did he scream optimistically? Did he shrug? Twitch his mouth?* I have to stop before I'm on the ground gasping for air.

Dr. Know-it-all calls me a few hours later (or what I like to call the two-week wait) to let me know that four follicles have caught up and we can continue with the protocol. I'm relieved— finally a bit of good news. I dance around my apartment to "Unstoppable" (Sia, 2016). "I'm unstoppable, I'm invincible, I'm so powerful, I'm so confident, yeah, I'm unstoppable today!

I have one more ultrasound a couple days later, and the follicles are all finally the right size. The smallest a follicle can be and still have a mature egg is 16 mm, but they like it to be between 18 and 22 mm. And yes, this drive is absolutely killing me. Thank you for asking.

Dr. Know-it-all instructs me to take the Ovidrel trigger shot at 8:00 p.m. and schedule my egg retrieval for thirty-six hours later. Katelin interviews Leo and a few other friends about their opinion of my journey and what I will be like as a mom. It is extremely touching to hear what my friends think about me. It's almost like hearing your own eulogy. People usually wait until you're dead to say these sentimental things.

Maybe this documentary is worth it. All women have mental breakdowns and lose their shit when it comes to infertility, right? Maybe? Not so much, but sometimes? Once in a while? In a blue moon?

Chapter 18
Growing Pains

Noah and I hike the long trek to Thousand Oaks. Of course, the rudeness in him stops to get breakfast when I'm not allowed to eat because of the anesthesia. I mean, come on, who doesn't like McDonald's breakfast? I really want hash browns. Soft on the inside, crunchy on the outside. Yummy goodness.

We arrive at Dr. Know-it-all's puppy mill, and of course, why would the anesthesiologist be covered under what I'd previously paid? I'm already in a shitty mood, and another $400 for fifteen minutes of anesthesia later, I'm in the surgical room while Noah pumps his gentleman's relish into a cup.

As I wake up, they guide Noah into the room. "All right, how are you doing, Lisa? Your husband is right here," declares the clueless nurse. Noah slowly creeps toward me to hold my hand but stares at the wall so he can't see the needle in the IV. I appreciate his efforts.

While I'm in the recovery area, the doctor lets me know he retrieved nine eggs. With all the bumps in the road, I'm amazed we got nine eggs.

Noah finds the nearest McDonald's and orders me hash browns. He guides me into my house and assists me into bed. He even walks my dogs. I sleep the rest of the day, hoping my dreams will become reality.

EASTER EGG HUNT

The egg retrieval is a minimally invasive fifteen-minute surgical procedure. No cuts, no stitches.

Your doctor will gently guide a needle attached to a catheter through the vaginal wall. One by one, eggs will be drawn out using light suction. They'll be collected in test tubes labeled with your name and unique identification numbers, and the tubes will be handed off to the embryologist. You'll be under sedation, so you won't feel a thing during the procedure.

The anesthesiologist will use a propofol-based anesthesia to ensure you feel no pain or discomfort. Legally, you can't drive yourself home after the process. I suggest not going to work afterward. Well, I guess you can go to work—just bring a lot of Tylenol. Like with any aesthesia, you will be slow moving and groggy. You'll even sign an agreement beforehand stating you will not drive or sign important documents for twenty-four hours. I fell asleep for hours once I got home.

You may experience soreness in the vaginal area, abdominal cramping, or spotting, all of which could last a few days. Tylenol will help. I like Tylenol—it cures all. #RhymeTime

Afterwards, the doctor will let you know how many eggs were retrieved.

The next day, the doctor will let you know how many matured and fertilized.

FERTILIZATION AND EMBRYO GROWTH

The next morning, I wait by the phone like any normal woman would do. Out of the nine eggs, only five were mature, and of those five, only four fertilized. The next update will be on day 3. It's nerve-racking; you just want confirmation that you're still in the game.

Fewer than half fertilized. I'm praying the numbers don't go to zero by day 3, as they keep decreasing. This process is worse than the two-week wait. You're on pins and needles waiting for the embryologist to see how many eggs are still alive.

On day 3, they tell me three of the four eggs are still growing and are now called a morula. Okay, whatever that means. At this point, I'm begging, pleading, saying Hail Marys. "Please let them get to day 5. Please, with sugar on top, sprinkles, and a cherry. *Please.*"

Day 5 comes, and two make it to blastocyst. Okay, at least I have two shots at pregnancy.

EMBRYOLOGIST, MY FIRST BABYSITTER

Following IVF insemination, culture dishes containing the sperm, eggs, and growth media are placed into an incubator, where the environmental conditions can be tightly controlled to mimic the conditions inside the woman's fallopian tubes and uterus. Over the next five days, the embryologist will monitor the embryos for fertilization and growth, reporting the progress. The embryologist follows each egg according to laboratory protocol, disturbing the forming embryo as little as possible to allow uninterrupted growth and maturation. Oh, so *that's* why they don't call me every day?

Day 0: Day of retrieval; insemination and ICSI only.

Day 1: Fertilization numbers are reported to the doctor.

Day 2: No observation.

Day 3: Growth check and assessment for transfer (now called a morula.)

Day 4: No observation.

Day 5: Growth check and assessment for transfer (now called a blastocyst).

The doctor jogs my memory, saying that due to my age—in case I forgot how old I was—we will biopsy the blastocysts and send the samples for preimplantation genetic selection (PGS) testing to check for any chromosomal abnormalities. It takes ten days to get the results. I am quickly learning "All you need is just a little patience." PGS testing is recommended for mothers of advanced maternal age (over thirty-five), as the likelihood of abnormalities increases after that age. I think this is mean—advanced maternal age? I guess it's better than calling it a geriatric pregnancy, which some doctors do.

Female age	Risk of a live birth with any chromosomal abnormality
25	1/476
30	1/385
35	1/164
40	1/51
45	1/15

BIOPYSING BABY

Cells are removed from an embryo for genetic testing before transferring it to the uterus.

Preimplantation genetic diagnosis (PGD) involves removing a cell from an IVF embryo to test for a specific genetic condition, such as cystic fibrosis, Tay-Sachs disease, muscular dystrophy, sickle cell anemia, or other genetic diseases for which the parents might be carriers. PGD tests for inherited diseases.

For example, if the male partner and female partner are both carriers of a recessive disease (such as cystic fibrosis), their child (conceived naturally) would have a 25 percent chance of having this horrible disease.

By having IVF and PGD, they can have "normal" embryos transferred so (if IVF is successful) their child won't have cystic fibrosis.

Preimplantation genetic screening (PGS) is the proper term for testing for overall chromosomal normalcy in embryos. PGS is not looking for a specific disease; it is screening the chromosomes for a copy number. If there's an extra chromosome, it's called a trisomy. For example, trisomy 21 is Down syndrome. If it is missing a chromosome, it's called a monosomy. A monosomy example is Turner syndrome; with this disorder, a female is born with only one X chromosome.

In theory, by testing the chromosomes of the embryos available for transfer, we can discard embryos with abnormal chromosomal arrangements and choose the embryo(s) for transfer from those with normal chromosomes.

I paid $1,100 dollars to see a genetic counselor for this exact information. You are welcome.

Tidbit: Most of us don't know there are *lots* of genetic disorders for which you may be a carrier. I highly suggest you and your partner do genetic screening through an outside lab. I used Counsyl. Each doctor may have a personal preference. I found that I'm a carrier of GSD-V, which is a metabolic disorder caused by an inability to break down complex sugar. Fortunately, Noah is not a carrier.

PGD FOR CARRIERS OF
CHROMOSMAL TRANSLOCATIONS

This is a rare situation in which a couple knows one of them has a chromosomal arrangement called a balanced translocation. When someone has a balanced chromosomal translocation, they are normal until they try to have a child.

When the chromosomes in their sperm or eggs join with those of their partner in a fertilized embryo, they have a high percentage of chromosomal abnormalities.

These embryos are at very high risk for miscarriage or could result in a child with birth defects. Transferring a PGS-normal embryo reduces this risk.

RISK WITHOUT PGS TESTING

The natural selection process prevents implantation of abnormal embryos. The large majority of chromosomally abnormal embryos will arrest in early development and not survive long enough to implant in the uterus. Some will implant and result in early miscarriages. An extremely small percentage can continue further into pregnancy and could progress to a live birth of a chromosomally abnormal baby.

Testing can be done in early pregnancy. There are noninvasive screening tests, such as blood tests or ultrasound evaluation of the baby. There is also invasive testing in early pregnancy, such as chorionic villus sampling (CVS) or amniocentesis. CVS is done at about 11–12 weeks of pregnancy. Amniocentesis can be done at about 16–18 weeks.

The overall risk for a chromosomally abnormal live birth does not appear to be increased by having IVF or IVF with ICSI.

GRADING, BLASTOCYSTS, EMBRYOS, OH MY!

Grading of embryo quality in the IVF lab can help pick the chromosomally normal embryos for transfer. Embryos that are "graded" on the higher end of the scale have lower rates of chromosomal abnormalities, compared to those embryos having lower grades.

Embryos that make normal-looking blastocysts on day 5 have lower rates of chromosomal abnormalities, compared to those embryos that do not make blastocysts (day 2 or 3 morulas).

Women of advanced reproductive age, or what I like to call sophisticated reproduction (thirty-eight or older), will sometimes have a very high percentage of chromosomally abnormal eggs.

Rather than using their own eggs, many of these women will need to do IVF with egg donation. Because egg donors are young (usually under thirty) and chromosomally abnormal eggs are much less common in young women, PGS is generally not used with donor eggs. Health class was never this complicated. You thought it was as simple as putting a P in the V? Ha! You're a funny one.

HOW MUCH WILL THIS SET YOU BACK?

The Good: Although they're expensive technologies, costs for PGS and PGD have been dropping over the years. No embryos were harmed in the making of this book.

The Bad: There will often need to be a frozen embryo transfer cycle done after PGD or PGS testing. You will have to wait another cycle, which again takes longer. It delays the process a little while longer, and we all know how much we love to wait.

The Ugly: About $3,500–$7,000, plus all other IVF costs. There are costs associated with the embryo biopsy procedure itself and for the genetics laboratory performing the genetic studies on the cells.

EMBRYO GRADING LOWDOWN

The day after egg retrieval, the new embryos will be checked for fertilization but not graded. They will not be checked again until day 3, 4, or 5 (blastocyst), depending on when the transfer was planned. On that day, the embryologist will check each embryo, "grade" it, pick the best for transfer, and determine if the remaining ones are suitable for freezing (cryopreservation).

DAY 3 EMBRYO

Grading of a day 3 embryo is based on the number of cells making up an embryo, the amount of fragmentation, and the symmetry of each of the embryo's cells (blastomeres).

A "perfect" day 3 embryo should be eight cells: no fragmentation, and all the cells are equal and symmetrical. Even very experienced embryologists can only reasonably "estimate" the chances for a successful pregnancy. Any good embryologist will tell you that "even though an embryo(s) looks good, it doesn't mean it is good" and vice versa. You gotta love science. By the end of this, you will be a pro or, at the very least, know what the hell your doctors are talking about.

BLASTOCYST

Scoring blastocysts is similar, but is has a completely different set of scoring criteria.

1. Blastocyst quality is determined by evaluating the outer ring of cells, known as the trophectoderm or trophoblastic cells, that will eventually form the placenta.
2. The inner cell mass (ICM), is made up of the stem cells in which the baby will develop.
3. The degree of expansion of the blastocyst cavity and whether or not it has started to "hatch" or break out of zona pellucida (shell). Don't worry: if you need a refresher, there's a glossary in the back of the book.

Expansion grade	Blastocyst development and stage status
1	Blastocoel cavity less than half the volume of the embryo
2	Blastocoel cavity more than half the volume of the embryo
3	Full blastocyst, cavity completely filling the embryo
4	Expanded blastocyst, cavity larger than the embryo, with thinning of the shell
5	Hatching out of the shell
6	Hatched out of the shell

ICM grade	Inner cell mass quality
A	Many cells, tightly packed
B	Several cells, loosely grouped
C	Very few cells

TE grade	Trophectoderm quality
A	Many cells, forming a cohesive layer
B	Few cells, forming a loose epithelium
C	Very few large cells

Blastocysts are given a quality grade for each of the three components, and the score is expressed with the expansion grade listed first, the inner cell mass grade listed second, and the trophectoderm grade listed third.

For example, a blastocyst quality grade of 4AB means that the blastocyst is expanded (grade 4), has many tightly packed cells in the inner cell mass (grade A), and has a trophectoderm with few cells forming a loose epithelium (grade B).

There are other blastocyst grading systems that use more letter grades than the Gardner system. For example, some clinics give component cells grades of D or even E in addition to the A, B, and C grades described above.

Blastocyst embryo grading is helpful. However, the potential of the embryo to continue normal development, implant, and result in a healthy baby being born is difficult to predict based on grading alone.

Like scoring day 3 embryos, scoring blastocysts is an imperfect science, and sometimes even very nice-looking blastocysts do not produce a pregnancy, whereas less-than-optimum ones do. Statistically, a very nice blastocyst has a greater chance of producing an ongoing pregnancy than a lesser-quality one. Again with all these contradictions!

A traumatic and/or bloody, difficult transfer can result in decreased pregnancy rates by disrupting the endometrial lining, introducing blood into the uterine cavity, triggering an inflammatory reaction, or having the embryos exposed to the outside environment (as opposed to the incubator environment) for too long.

Several months before an embryo transfer, a mock transfer can be done to measure the depth of the uterine cavity and the ease or difficulty of eventual embryo transfer so there won't be any surprises at the time of the actual embryo transfer. While doing a mock transfer, an endometrial receptivity analysis (ERA) test is done by sampling a small amount of endometrial tissue. This will determine if the endometrium is receptive or not, establishing the best day for transferring the embryo. ERA test findings have indicated 20–25 percent of embryo transfers are happening too early or too late. Embryo transfers take less than thirty seconds from the time the embryos are removed from the culture environment of the incubator to the time they're loaded in the transfer catheter. A steady hand wins the race.

Ten days later, I receive a call informing me I have one normal (euploid) and one abnormal (aneuploid). The aneuploid is missing one of its number 22 chromosomes, but it's mosaic. Mosaicism can complicate matters. An embryo is a mosaic if there are two (or more) different chromosomal patterns in the cells of that embryo. There is evidence mosaic embryos sometimes "self-repair" or possibly designate abnormal cells preferentially to the placenta instead of the fetus. More research on mosaicism is needed. The question becomes: Can these mosaic embryos self-correct in the uterus and become a normal, healthy baby?

The doctor isn't going to volunteer the sexes, but I ask because I am impatient, and I find out the normal one is a boy, and the abnormal one is a girl. Due to this ever-evolving information, I have my "mosaic" embryo frozen, waiting for further research.

Fun fact: Some countries will not reveal the gender, as gender selecting has been banned. Chrissy Teigen got tremendous amounts of flack because she chose a girl.

Chapter 19
Another Roadblock

I have never been so unbelievably ecstatic for Aunt Flo to show up! Time to get this baby in its buggy. I bounce my legs in the exam room waiting to talk to Doc Know-it-all, expecting to hear the plan to prep my lining for transfer. Instead, he informs me "University" hospital forgot an important test called a saline sonogram. Of course they did, and he needs to perform it before we move forward. Good news: he's willing to do it right now.

SALINE SONOGRAM LOWDOWN

A saline infusion sonohysterography (say that ten times fast), also called an SIS or saline ultrasound, is a test where a small volume of saline is inserted into the uterus, allowing the lining to be clearly seen on an ultrasound scan. They are looking for polyps, tumors, fibroids, and congenital malformations. While doing this test, many doctors biopsy the lining of the endometrium (uterus) to see if there is any inflammation that requires antibiotics.

This hurts almost as bad as the HSG test. (Later, I learn from my final doctor, it should be a painless procedure and only hurt when you have an unskilled doctor.) Turns out, a polyp is taking up valuable real estate in my uterus. Another setback. Rather than prepping for a frozen embryo transfer (FET), I'm getting authorization from my insurance for a polyp removal. The tech term is a hysteroscopy. Thank God this is considered medically necessary and not an out-of-pocket expense.

Unfortunately, another cycle goes by before beginning the FET prep. A few days before Christmas, I finally have an appointment to discuss the lining prep and transfer. The doctor prescribes estrogen and schedules a series of appointments over the next two and a half weeks to monitor my uterine lining and estrogen levels. I forget why. I think to check your estrogen levels so your body is ready for a transfer. The reason this is important is to simulate the changes that normally occur during a regular menstrual cycle, since your body isn't truly ovulating.

New year, new outlook. Transfer day! Leo accompanies me to a procedure room. The room is dark, lit only by the ultrasound machine. How can the doctor see what he's doing? Run for your life if this is your setup!

The doctor walks in and says, "Hello, Noah. It's nice to see you again." Oh, no, another sign my doctor runs a sweatshop. He doesn't even remember what his patients look like? If you met Leo and Noah, you would realize that they look absolutely, 100 percent, like polar opposites. Not even the same spectrum. Like, I'm talking two totally different races. C'mon, man!

The most uncomfortable part of this procedure is that you have to do it with a full bladder. My bladder isn't full enough, so they bring me two bottles of water and tell me to drink. I am tremendously impressed I don't pee on Dr. Know-it-all. He can thank me later. The transfer of the embryo is quick but more painful than expected, as he has trouble feeding the catheter through my cervix.

After the procedure, I have to lie there for fifteen minutes with my knees bent up. This feels like an eternity, since my bladder is about to explode. Just imagine you're on a car ride and you have to pee, but you can't go for an hour. The tension builds and builds, and all you can think about is flowing water, rain, and peeing. Mind over matter—nope, my urethra is tickling.

I go home and binge on Netflix. Opinions vary from doctor to doctor as to the level of activity you should have after a transfer.

Some say go back to life as normal, while others say two days of couch rest is necessary. I will always choose the latter, especially when a child is involved.

Chapter 20
The Loss of a Child

A few days later, I'm bedridden. My chest hurts, my throat hurts, and my head hurts. I can't move. I'm incredibly weak. For a minute, I think, *Is this what it's supposed to feel like?* I call the nurse, and she assures me that being sick won't affect the implantation; however, being sick can cause stress on the body, and stress can negatively affect implantation. Learning from past mistakes, I don't symptom spot. I wait ten days before I take my first pregnancy test. I don't want to take one at all, but alas, I break at the ten-day mark. It's negative, but I try to tell myself it's too early. I'm in my head: *It will work. You don't pay $20,000 for something not to work.* I'm not disappointed yet, but the "oh, shits" start popping into my head.

I take another test on day 13. Still negative. Maybe the hCG is low and these tests aren't sensitive enough. Although hope is dwindling, I still have faith the bloodwork will show levels of hCG, however low.

When I go to the fertility clinic, I'm greeted with smiles and optimism. The nurses and staff are supportive and hopeful that this is the one, as Dr. Know-it-all has had copious amounts of success. The girl takes my blood and scolds me for taking a test at home. She tells me not to give up and it's not over yet. I go home feeling a glimmer of hope.

It takes centuries for them to call me with the results. I'm surprised it isn't the doctor on the phone but one of his many nurses. I can immediately tell by the tone of her voice that it isn't good news. "I'm sorry, it is negative." It's unemotional, cold. She doesn't give a flying F. She's rushing to get off the phone when I ask if I can talk to the doctor. I grow upset and have to pull teeth to convince her to let me speak with the doctor. "Oh, no, sorry. We're done. See you later. Buh-bye." You'd think they'd be more helpful and want you to schedule an appointment to go over your next options. Although I predicted this result, I'm crushed and broken inside. My knees collapse from underneath me. "Why?" is all I could scream up at the heavens.

1/20/17

Should I give up? Should I not be a mom? Why was I being punished? Did I do something to deserve this? I couldn't be the only one putting myself in a corner.

I was completely convinced this was going to work. I bought an astronomical amount of boy clothes. I visualized my chubby cherub. I visualized a life with him. I was attached to him. His first day at school, playing sports, being Mama's little man. I was mentally fatigued by this struggle. I dismantled the crib and got rid of everything I had ever bought for the baby. Maybe I was jinxing myself by having it.

How could I pick myself up? Would I be able to move on? How does life go on when you have so much love to give and no one to share it with? I had never felt more alone than in that moment. The heaviness in my heart yearned for a child.

I spoke with Dr. Know-it-all about my sadness, and he gave me a list of recommended therapists who specialize in fertility. When I called one of the ladies, I told her I felt grief and disappointment, and she assured me it was normal to feel like someone had died after the failure of IVF. I was going through the stages of grief. She recommended I reach out to fertility support groups to process my emotions and find solidarity.

SOMEONE TO BLAME

I keep going back to how painful the transfer was. He had a hard time feeding the catheter through my cervix. Did he cause bleeding? Could blood have gotten into my uterus, causing inflammation? Was this a traumatic transfer? Was this the reason my boy didn't implant? I guess I will never know. I will never know what a life with Mama's little man would have been like.

Katelin finished her documentary, which earned her an A on her final. To this day, I have yet to view it because that period in my life is too upsetting to relive. I'm sure someday I will want to watch, just to remember what I went through. Who am I kidding? I never want to watch it. I never want to remember what I could have had and didn't get the chance. I never want to remember the carelessness of the doctor. The aloofness of the nurse. I never want to remember the money I wasted. The time I wasted. I never want to remember I could have had *my* own Cooper.

Chapter 21
I'm Not Alone

When I was beginning my journey, one tidbit Dr. Nameless told me was about a support group called Resolve. I haven't looked into this program, but after the devastating loss of the transfer, it's time to seek support and hopefully shed light on this trying time. I begin by browsing the Resolve website (resolve.org) for available meetings. I select a peer-led one; they also have other gatherings that are professionally led.

I go to one on Sunset Boulevard. People are gathered in the community room. I don't know what to expect. I'm nervous, but I go inside. To my surprise, it's not only women of "advanced maternal age." There are men and women of all ages and races. Infertility doesn't show prejudice.

As the discussion begins, I quickly realize that we all have different reasons to be there, but the struggle of infertility is changing us from strangers to friends. I'm surrounded by people who genuinely understand the emotional roller coaster I'm riding.

Even though I don't share my story, the comfort this group provides makes me feel safe. I love my family and friends, but up until now, I haven't talked to anyone who understands my anguish and frustration. I constantly receive generic responses: "Relax," "Take a vacation," "It will happen when you stop trying," "Get drunk and let it happen!" *Shut up!* No person going through a fertility journey wants to hear half-witted, half-brained, insensitive suggestions.

At the Resolve meeting, someone tells me about Facebook support groups to join. I begin my search with keywords and join every single group I can find—probably seventy-five. I'm neurotic, if you haven't figured that out already. These groups are filled with women going through the exact same situation and at different stages. You give advice about what you know and ask about what you don't. It's a give and take of information. There's a combination of success and horror stories. Some leave me inspired, while others increase my anxiety.

At first, all I do is observe. You quickly become attached to people's stories. These groups become my soul purpose for being on Facebook—chat rooms for the millennial age. You feel for people going through loss and then gain hope from success stories. I go on, wanting updates and fueling my passion. The more I learn, the more I become empowered about my own fertility. The knowledge makes me have control over the situation. I wish I had known about these groups at the beginning of my journey instead of nearing the end. Or at least I think it's the end.

Every once in a great while, someone will post a baby picture chronicling their journey and triumphant success story.

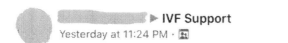

IVF Support ...
Yesterday at 11:24 PM ·

I post this as hope for every one here I have been apart of this group many years have had 3 iui all negitive 2 retrivals and 5 transfers a hysterscopy, ERA, 3 miscarriages been told by my doctor i need a suroggot twice well I had my ivf miracles on 4/10 35 weeks but perfect in every way I still can't say it without crying but I'm a mom don't give up

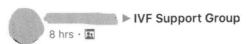

▶ IVF Support Group

8 hrs ·

Ladies , I wanted everyone to know and be strong because it can happen. I had a miscarriage in 2013 , then in 2015 I had a fibroid and an ovary removed along with cysts. My husband was found with low morphology and I had a low count in my remaining ovary. But with faith and a lot of support from you ladies, my husband and I via emergency c- section meet out little prince this past Wednesday.

Please meet ▓▓▓▓▓, our little perfect miracle. We are in love and couldn't be more grateful, thankful and over the moon to have him with us .

These reignite my flame to keep fighting for my baby. Okay, I'm not going to give up on motherhood, which I am so passionate about. I am meant to be a mom. I am meant to give love.

FACEBOOK IVF SUPPORT GROUPS

IVF Support

IVF Support 36+

IVF with PGD/PGS Support Group

IUI TTC Support Group

Clomid, Femara, IVF & Infertility

IUI & IVF Support Health Group

IUI & IVF Support Loss Group

TTC/Pregnancy Over 35

Single Mothers by Choice

IVF Support Group

IVF Pregnancy Support

IUI & IVF Support

IVF Journey

IVF TTC Baby #1

IVF or Poor Responders

IVF Egg Donors

Infertility Support Group

Operation Find the Storks

Egg Donor Angels Recipients Only Support Group

IUI & IVF Support Pregnancy Group

Sock Buddies Infertility (IVF, IUI, ICSI, FET)

Operation Find the Storks is a page dedicated to the search and retrieval of LuLaRoe stork leggings in either purple or black. By the way, ladies, those are the only two colors. Facebook legend has it that once you get these hard-to-find stork pants, a baby will find its way to you. I thought, *What the heck. I'll join.* After I share my story in a few posts, a woman named Marissa from Idaho decides to gift the leggings to me, as she just gave birth to her baby boy. Yes, I'm buying into the bullshit, okay? I got the leggings. I'm getting that baby!

Sock Buddies Infertility is a support group that highlights all infertility topics and where woman gift other women fertility socks for good luck. What are fertility socks, you ask? They have cute quotes—"IVF got this," "You are Strong" (with pictures of sperm on the toes), "Fierce," "Hope," and other positive affirmations—and women wear them to their insemination or embryo transfer. I'm so proud of women—we've literally thought of everything.

Chapter 22
Running Out of Time

It's been one year since I kicked off this voyage. I'm flat broke, but where there's a will, there's a way. Cliché, but that's what keeps me going. One tube is open, so rather than doing nothing while I save up, I elect to attempt the old-fashioned way of timed-by-ovulation kits.

I summon Noah to discuss my dilemma. I am completely out of money, but I don't want to concede.

"I don't even know what to do anymore." My voice thickens.

"Well, is there any chance you can get pregnant naturally?" Noah lightly strokes my shoulder.

"It's a small chance, but miracles happen."

"Let's just do that!"

"Did you not understand me? I have no money."

"No, I heard you. I want to do this for you. You don't have to pay me." My heart seems to freeze and pound at the same time. There is no reason for him to do this for me.

I can't contain my excitement. I embrace Noah and press my lips against his with no deflection. He wraps his arms around me, not letting go. I'm not doing it alone anymore. I have never felt more determined.

Over the next six months, the meetings for baby dancing become more than a quick wham-bam. We cook dinners, talk for hours, and cuddle while watching documentaries. Noah and I go to the movies and museums and dance the night away. We become inseparable friends, and I do what no woman should ever do in my state: I fall in love with him. The way he gazes at me, I believe he is too.

It starts like any normal outing at Westwood's 800 Degrees pizzeria. He grins at me, which pours shivers down my spine. I know this is the moment I've been waiting for. The sign I need to know everything is going to be okay.

"I'm so glad the baby is going to have your genes," I say.

"Why?" he questions.

"You're perfect."

"I'm not perfect. I hate when you say that. It makes me feel uncomfortable," he snaps back.

"But to me, you're perfect. I love you," I divulge. Probably not the most opportune time, but it comes out, and I have to live with it.

"I have love for you, but it's not a romantic love, and it never will be." My chest gets tight, color drains from my face, and I swallow hard. My body becomes lifeless. I'm humiliated. His response wounds my spirit. I'm completely confused. Why would he do this for me without a motive? (That is according to Leo—he said he wouldn't do this for anyone.) Don't listen to your friends, because it will do your head in and you'll say the three inappropriate words not meant to be uttered.

He leans toward me. I extend my arm and say, "Don't. Leave." He snatches the to-go box and disappears past the doors and into the dusk. A feeling of unworthiness washes over me. I stare blankly at nothing. The ambience blurs together. I'm paralyzed. What the hell did I do? *Why can't you ever just shut your mouth, Lisa?* The waiter checks on me. I'm blank. No words come out of my mouth. I'm a statue—slumped shoulders, limp posture. I don't know how long I remain here, but my heart breaks today.

After the blowup with Noah, the only way to continue this relationship, or what is left of it, is to do an IUI, because that's only a thousand dollars. I can no longer be intimate with him.

Leo and I grab coffee, and I explain how I fell for Noah. "This is ridiculous. It's the medicine. You are not in love. You are an emotional basket case. He's just been there for you in your time of need. Of course you feel attached and vulnerable. He's seen you at your worst and stuck by you."

I'm enraged, "That's not true." I don't want it to be true, but I know it is. All the hormones, sex, and late-night chats into the morning—how could I not be in love? How could it not be a relationship?

"I don't want you to keep doing timed intercourses with him. You'll fall deeper and may not be able to pick yourself back up."

I throw my hands up in the air. "Well, what am I supposed to do then, huh?"

"Lisa, he has his own life. He's dating other women."

"You don't know that."

"Don't be ridiculous, Lisa."

We sit there in silence as I let those words sink in. "What am I supposed to do? I don't have money for IVF!"

"Well, how much is an IUI?"

"About a thousand dollars, but I don't even have that."

"Let me lend it to you. You need to stop the intimacy."

As much as I want to do this, I feel pressure as the debt keeps mounting. Leo tells me never to worry about the money. Happiness has no price tag. Money should never be the reason you can't do something. It shouldn't be a hindrance. I finally agree and feel a little weight lifted off my shoulders for the time being.

I suck it up and text Noah. I apologize for my outburst and, once again, blame it on the hormones. He tells me he never wants to hurt me. "I've only ever been in love once. It's not you. I don't know if I will ever find someone with all the attributes I am looking for." *What are you looking for?* I think. *Stop it, Lisa! Baby, baby, baby, baby. Blah, blah, blah. Noah's on board. I'm not his type, meh, meh, meh.*

The IUI doesn't work. During the WTF meeting with Dr. Know-it-all, he says, "It's been a year since we first met, and from day one I told you IVF is your only option. On top of that, your reserve has depleted even further, and I don't expect I would get more than five eggs." I have a truthful and transparent conversation with him about my finances. He seems sympathetic, as this is his practice. He makes the rules. He offers me a reduced rate and payment plan. As grateful as I am, how am I even going to get the money for the down payment and medication? I'm sounding like a Debbie Downer, and I shouldn't be. I know I'm not alone in my feelings. Most people stress over trying to find the money for treatments. Once again, Leo, my savior, volunteers to front me the money. As grateful as I am, I feel horrible because this isn't his responsibility.

Dr. Know-it-all tells me I would get half the amount of eggs. He adds the human growth hormone Omnitrope to my protocol, which is what they give short kids to grow. On all the websites and support groups, this is supposed to soup up your eggs. After all, it costs $1,000 for three vials. Can you imagine? This better work.

Egg retrieval day commences, and Dr. Know-it-all only obtains four eggs. I'm not upset, because I trust this medication to improve the egg quality.

Dr. Know-it-all calls the next day with devastating news: none of my eggs fertilized. He doesn't give a rat's ass—no compassion and ruthless. Even though I only made it to retrieval, he still makes me pay for the cost of the embryologist work, IVF lab, prepping for transfer, and frozen embryo transfer. I mean, I'm grateful for the payment plan, but why am I responsible for treatments he didn't perform? As I mentioned, he owns the practice. Why is he being apathetic? Before he hangs up, he tells me the only way I can become pregnant is with donor eggs. Woah, what? As if he couldn't be even more of a dick. Thank you for taking away my womanhood in one sharp kick. I throw my phone against the wall. Fuck him! Fuck him and his cattle ranch! Fuck him and his narcissistic personality! I pace the room with purpose. I seize a pillow from the couch, bury my face, and belt out the shrillest blood-curdling scream.

After the cheerful tête-à-tête with Dr. Egotistical Asshole, my first phone call isn't to Leo; it's to Noah. I can accept the loss of my genetics, but I don't want to lose his. Right on cue, he says I can count on him. He pays his condolences and bolsters me by saying he isn't going anywhere. He is devoted to my pregnancy battle, and so am I. How could you not love him?

I wish I knew about egg freezing. Was it even around in my early twenties? If I can give any advice to young girls reading this, please freeze your eggs as soon as possible. Although you can freeze your eggs at any time, for the best quality and quantity of eggs, I suggest doing it during your early to mid-twenties.

Tidbit: If you work for Apple or Facebook, they will cover the $10,000 cost for freezing your eggs. Check with your own insurance, as you never know. A round of egg freezing can cost between $7,000 and $12,000, plus additional fees for storage and drugs.

Chapter 23
Third Time's the Charm

Most women go through a period when they grieve the loss of their own genetics. I've read stories where women take six months or more to accept the news and move forward using donor eggs. I never experience this. No matter where the eggs come from, this will be my baby.

My egg retrieval is on October 11th, and I discover the news on October 12th. I am motivated to be a mom. I set up a consultation for IVF with donor eggs on November 6th. I do extensive research this time to find the perfect doctor. I acquire the doctor who is the go-to guy for national TV shows, including *Dr. Oz, Dr. Phil, The Doctors, Good Morning America*, and *The Today Show*. He is a pioneer in egg freezing and donor egg cycles.

Amidst all the darkness, a ray of light shines down. Following a seven-year battle with Worker's Comp over my back injury, I receive my settlement payment. Is this divine intervention? Not only can I clear out my fertility debts, I actually have the money to move forward with donor IVF.

The minute I walk into the Santa Monica office, I'm in utopia. I squeeze Noah's arm eagerly. The energy is calm and serene. The woman at the counter speaks in a soft voice. I'm the only one in the waiting room. With Dr. Know-it-all, I had gotten accustomed to lobbies with twenty women and waiting areas in the back by exam rooms. The new clinic focuses on the individual patient and personalized care rather than running a sweatshop.

The hallways are adorned with awards, copies of articles he's written for medical journals, and still photos of him on television shows. I proceed into a small meeting room, where there are celebrity pictures with thank-you notes praising Dr. John Jain for helping them create their child. What I've wanted all along.

Dr. Jain stands tall with his shoulders back as he glides into the room. There is an instant warmth. He is confident without being smug. He doesn't have my medical records; he spends a good chunk of time asking questions and building a medical history profile for us. He's realistic about issues. He asks Noah if he does drugs. Noah responds sheepishly, "Well, I smoke weed."

Without hesitation, Dr. Jain says, "That's okay. There's no real evidence that marijuana affects sperm count." Noah engages with Dr. Jain about our history.

Dr. Jain concludes, "There is really nothing you can do outside medical treatments to conceive."

Okay, there is nothing I can do on my own to change this outcome? So, worrying is out of the question now. Noah puts his arm around me and tells Dr. Jain, "I wish we had met you first. I've been telling her she needs to relax." We agree with Dr. Jain to move forward with donor egg IVF.

Sarah, a pretty blonde in her early thirties, greets us with a compassionate smile. She goes over pricing, and I decide on a shared fresh cycle guaranteeing eight healthy mature eggs. I open up my checkbook and cringe as I write out the $29,800 check. She literally says, which I think is reckless, "I can almost guarantee your journey ends here."

Chapter 24
Am I Shallow?

WHERE DO I BEGIN? I'M 5'5".
SHOULD MY DONOR BE 5'9" OR 5'11"?

Sifting through the national frozen-egg-donor databases, I am immediately advised by Sarah that frozen eggs should *never* be shipped. I'm not finding a suitable donor there anyway. Sarah suggests I look at their in-house donors for a fresh cycle.

Dr. Jain's database has a whole new caliber of donors. The best of the best. The cream of the crop. The crème de la crème. Whatever ethnicity or search filters you choose results in highly educated, stunning women with a excess of artistic and athletic abilities. Not only do their profiles read like college applications; they provide more information than a high-end dating site. Am I choosing a donor or a best friend? Their pictures were all pulled from Instagram, obviously. You can tell these women had professional photos taken and put their best pictures up like they would on a dating profile. Well, considering they are making $8,000 a pop, they should step up their game. A red-light district window flashing, "Pick me, pick me!" Am I shallow for wanting a gorgeous donor?

Donor #7537 Extended Profile

Height	Weight (lbs.)	Ethnic Origin	Hair Color	Eye Color
5'7"	125	Caucasian	Blonde	Blue

Freckles:	Dimples:	Acne Problems:	Birthmarks:
Yes	No	No	No

Body Type/Build:	Native Language:	Do you speak other languages?	Which languages?
Slim	English	Yes	French, Spanish
Favorite Sport	**Favorite Music**	**Athletic Ability**	**Artistic Skills and Creativity**
Surfing	Rock, folk	Surfing, soccer, track and field	Filmmaking, photography, writing
Musical Abilities	**Other Special Talents**	**Favorite Color**	**Favorite Food**
Piano, guitar	Creative design	Turquoise	Vegan pasta

Education	High School	Undergrad/College	Masters/PhD
Completed?	Yes	Yes	No
Major	General	Environmental Science	
GPA	4.3	3.8	

Describe your personality and character: (A generic answer everyone would ever say about themselves.)

What would you say is your strongest personal trait? Why? Optimistic. I see the good in every circumstance. (Isn't she the sweetest?)

How do you think others would describe you? Humble, dependable, honest, driven, kind. (You know, the usual.)

Describe yourself as a child (personality, health, and happiness): I was a very active child. (And a ton of other amazing things that any child would love doing.)

What was it like growing up in your family? (Of course, she said it wasn't always easy, but she wouldn't change it for the world.)

124

Where would you most like to travel and why? Tahiti. (And she brings it back to surfing and ocean and island. Hippie.)

Have you had any unique travel experiences that you feel have helped shape your way of thinking? (She volunteered in Nepal. Talking about how she worked in these impoverished communities yet seeing how happy they are.)

Please describe any unique educational experiences you have had: I went to UC Berkley. (Blah, blah, blah. She's super smart.)

What is your philosophy on life? Embrace the present. (Who is this chick? Is she, like, the Dalai Lama?)

What is your ultimate goal and ambition in life? To live presently, create consciously, heal humanity through my art. (I guess she is.)

Why do you want to be an egg donor? My motivation to donate my eggs stems from my love for life and family. (I always wonder what motivates someone to do this, other than money.)

Academic societies, awards, scholarships, organizations, and extracurricular activities: (Editor of the school newspaper, student of the world, multiple science awards.)

I ponder for a minute, and I realize I'm buying genetic material, so shouldn't I buy the best? After all, she needs to look like Noah would sleep with her. I pick a 5'7" chick with blonde hair, green eyes, and a perfectly toned body. She is college educated, creative, and athletic. She states she has never had facial plastic surgery, but bitch, please—those lips are faker than a Real Housewife, which makes me think, *Is she college educated? Does she know what facial plastic surgery means? Or does she think an enhancement filler doesn't count?*

As I select a donor, Sarah explains to me (numerous times) that the child comes out looking like the birth mother. How is this possible? "Epigenetics," she swoons. I'm listening. Epigenetics for beginners: although the DNA will be from the egg and sperm donors, my DNA will cause genes to be turned off or on. This is what makes us unique. It controls hair color, skin color, taste in foods, and personality. How can I make my DNA choose certain ones? My body will determine which ones get turned on or off and encourage traits similar to my own to be expressed. My baby better have my flipping, flowing auburn locks!

The clinic reaches the "prized possession" to find out when she will be open to cycle next. Luckily, she is available now and stoked about her first donation.

A lot of legality goes into egg donation. I'm put into contact with a third-party reproductive lawyer, and for $750, he draws up the necessary agreements for all parties involved. To be precise, mine is eighteen pages. I would put it in for you, but it might be outdated—or that is a ridiculous number of pages to put in the book, one of the two.

KEY POINTS YOU NEED TO KNOW ABOUT YOUR FERTILITY AND EGG DONATION AGREEMENT

1.3 Donor will give eggs in exchange for payment.

1.5 Even though the law is evolving in California and elsewhere, Donor and Intended Parent agree the Intended Parent will have sole legal custody. Donor has no custody, including visitation, parental, or financial obligations of any kind or claims to the Child.

1.6 In the event the Donor is married (or is in a domestic partnership relationship), the Donor's husband or registered domestic partner shall be included as a party to this Agreement.

Tidbit: Because they are married, her eggs are like joint property.

1.7 California Family Code section 7613 remains unsettled at this time. Therefore, Donor and Intended Parent(s) agree to accept the inescapable legal risks inherent in egg donation, including the risks one or more persons may not comply with the terms of this Agreement or related agreements; the laws could be changed to interfere with the Parties' intentions; and parental rights of egg donors and egg recipients are subject to unknown interpretation by the courts.

Tidbit: This one freaked me out, because after talking with the lawyer, I found out no one has won a custody case in sixteen years. That means that although we have this agreement, if the laws change to interfere with the parties' intentions, it would be up to the court to decide who has the rights to the child. I would hunt a bitch down and potentially end up in jail if that happened to me. I'm just saying, don't mess with me!

1.8 Donor waives all parental rights and responsibilities to any Child conceived with the use of the eggs retrieved from her body.

1.9 Intended Parent(s) shall be conclusively presumed to be the legal parent(s) of any Child(ren) conceived pursuant to this Agreement.

2.0 All anonymity of both Parties' personal and medical information remains private.

3.1 Donor has given accurate medical information to the best of her knowledge.

3.2 Donor agrees to take all medications prescribed by Doctor. *Very important!*

3.3 Donor represents she has or will undergo a psychological assessment.

3.4 Donor agrees she will not participate in dangerous sports or activities, smoke cigarettes or use any other tobacco products, drink alcohol to excess, use any illegal drugs, or use any non-prescription drugs or medication without prior approval of the Physician. Smoking affects egg maturation.

3.7 Except for money or insurance proceeds payable to Donor, she holds Intended Parent(s) hold harmless. She can't go after Intended Parents for any complications suffered during the procedures performed or any pain, suffering, or psychological conditions resulting from donation.

3.8 Native American Indian Ancestry. Donor represents neither she nor any living and/or deceased member of her immediate or extended family is and/or ever has been a registered member of any Native American Indian or Alaskan Indian tribe.

Tidbit: there have been cases of egg and sperm donations done by persons of these ancestries in which the tribe has claimed custody of the resulting children and won!

4.1 Intended Parent(s) release Donor from any legal, financial, and moral responsibility whatsoever for the Child, whether or not the Child develops abnormally.

4.2 Intended Parent(s) are aware of the risk pregnancy may result in genetic and congenital abnormalities.

4.3 Intended Parent(s) payment to fertility clinic will pay for laboratory costs, physician fees, and expenses for egg removal.

4.4 Donor should receive a sum of $8,000. Reimbursement is not allowed to get paid for eggs, so they phrase it differently.

Tidbit: also, some egg donors could ask for more money.

4.5 If Donor cancels cycle, she will only get $500.*

*This is important because if she cancels, you are not obligated to pay the full amount.

4.6 Neither the fertility clinic nor Intended Parent(s) shall be liable for Donor's lost wages.

4.7 Money that went to the Donor is managed by the fertility clinic.

5.1 Donor acknowledges a Child created with Donor's donated eggs may, in the future, seek out additional information about Donor. However, Donor's identity and/or any information that may reasonably lead to the disclosure of the Donor's identity shall not be provided to the Child without the Intended Parents' and Donor's prior written consent.

5.2 Keep fertility clinic up to date on address, illness, or death for both Parties.

5.3 In the future, should it become necessary to give or obtain additional medical information concerning Donor and such Child or Children, the Parties hereby agree to use best efforts to inform SMF of any and all changes in the contact information for such Party.

5.4 If you want to contact the other party, you must go through the fertility clinic first.

5.5 If we have to go to court, we release fertility clinic of any costs, liability, or obligations. Although the Child is genetically related to Donor and Intended Parent(s), Child will be considered a "child of marriage" of Intended Parents. Pursuant to California Family Code section 7613(b).

5.6 Donor and Intended Parent(s) acknowledge and agree egg donation is a new medical technology with both known and unknown medical, psychological, legal, and other risks to all participants.

5.7 No guarantee of a live child, free of birth defects or other ailments, conditions, or illnesses.

6.0 Hold Fertility clinic harmless for *everything*.

7.0 At any time prior to the active preparation for egg retrieval, either Party may terminate this Agreement effective upon two days' prior written notice to the other Party.

8.0 All standard contract provisions (which was another two to three pages).

Ask your fertility clinic if they have any recommendations for lawyers or lawyers they work with. If not, when searching online, look for a lawyer who specializes in third-party reproduction law.

Chapter 25
Acupuncture!

Dr. Jain tells me to do acupuncture to help prep my lining. I'm up for anything and everything to make my pregnancy a success.

First and foremost, you should look for an acupuncturist who specializes in fertility (and preferably has a PhD). I go to Dr. Alex Ezzati. He is kind, compassionate, and also a little too good-looking for my taste. His office is welcoming and Zen-like. The examination rooms are dimly lit with crystal lamps, and soothing meditation music surrounds me. He begins my treatments by having me eliminate gluten and reduce dairy. Additionally, he asks me to buy royal jelly and eat a teaspoon of it every day. Royal jelly—I'll say it again—tastes like bitter shit. I try mixing it with honey in the teaspoon, but it barely covers up the staleness.

Going into acupuncture, I think it's kind of hocus pocus. When I meet Dr. Alex, he does a thorough examination, like a doctor would. He decides to incorporate other physical ailments into my fertility treatment.

I'm worried this treatment will be like tiny daggers poking me. After he inserts a few needles without my noticing, I thank my good graces it doesn't hurt. I look like Hellraiser, but I feel like a Disney character floating on an imaginary cloud. Certain points cause an electrical pulsating feeling to run down my leg. That's how I know it's working.

He places needles from the top of my head to my toes and leaves them there for twenty minutes. He takes them out, I roll over on my back, and he does it again. If anything, I'm using this time to clear my head and get my mind off the anxiety. Getting rid of my negative thoughts. Getting rid of all my worries. Getting rid of the utter crap of day-to-day life and being present in this moment. I focus on being pregnant. Focus on the joy of motherhood. Focus on love. When I leave his office, I feel more relaxed, and the stress seems to go away.

I go once a week, and after a few weeks, I notice physical differences. I no longer have back pain, and my anxiety has disappeared. I didn't know I could feel this way again. I've had back pain for seven years, and now it's vanished. I don't need pain meds anymore. Euphoria fills my body. I'm light as a feather, and my mind is clear. I'm dancing on rainbows—and no, I'm not on hallucinogens.

Dr. Alex becomes a friend and advocate in my fertility. It's more than a job for him. He wants a triumphant victory for me.

THE MOXA EXPERIENCE

As the donor-egg IVF transfer nears, Dr. Alex begins incorporating mugwort herb (moxa) into my treatment. Moxa is burned in different ways, with the intention of bringing heat to the area being treated. Mugwort is known to stimulate blood flow to the pelvic area, especially to the uterus. Moxa therapy involves lighting yourself on fire—well, almost. It involves placing the herb on specific points on your body and lighting it on fire, but without burning yourself. Such a trickster I am—you have to have a sense of humor!

Disclaimer: Just kidding—it doesn't burst into flames. It burns like incense. Still, leave this to the professionals, folks!

WHY AND HOW ACUPUNCTURE HELPS

Begin treatments as early as possible and maintain a consistent treatment schedule. Results generally take at least three menstrual cycles; however, even a single treatment can be very beneficial by reducing your stress and encouraging calm introspection.

INFERTILITY

Traditional Chinese medicine works by regulating your hormonal imbalances to bring your body toward optimum health through the use of nutritional counseling, herbal medicine, and acupuncture. Please speak with your reproductive endocrinologist, as mine didn't want me taking any herbs. These techniques help enhance fertility by balancing your endocrine, nervous, and immune systems, and they give your body the ability to achieve conception.

Certain foods and supplements will assist in creating favorable conditions for reproductive health.

Fertility challenges and hormonal imbalances are linked to the endocrine and reproductive systems (which are closely tied to your ovaries) and to the hypothalamus and pituitary glands in your brain. These systems are responsible for menstruation, menopause, and ovulation. Together, these make up the hypothalamic-pituitary-ovarian axis (HPO). The HPO is delicately balanced and can easily be thrown out of equilibrium by stress, the aging process, or any number of other factors. Acupuncture has been proven to regulate the HPO, optimizing its ability to function properly, which subsequently will increase your chances of conception. Patients report they have a much better sense of well-being, greater energy, and less depression and anxiety when they receive acupuncture treatments.

Research shows acupuncture can increase the success of IVF procedures by 27–43 percent—a good enough statistic for me!

Acupuncture reduces the side effects of the medications. These side effects range from hot flashes and mood swings to gas, bloating, and other digestive disturbances. I wish I'd known that when I was taking the disastrous Clomid! It also increases blood flow to your uterus, thereby thickening the endometrial lining and preparing it for implantation.

EMBRYO TRANSFER

You will do acupuncture before and after the day of the transfer. Studies show this can increase your chances of achieving pregnancy by reducing stress, relaxing the uterus, and reducing cramping.

ELEVATED FSH

Higher FSH levels are a perfectly normal function of aging but are problematic for conception. Acupuncture may help decrease FSH levels. This is important because your FSH levels are often an indicator of how well you will respond to IVF treatment. They indicate poor ovarian reserve, premature ovarian aging, or declining ovarian reserve.

STRESS

Studies show women with high stress levels are up to 93 percent less likely to conceive. Stress not only reduces blood flow to your reproductive organs but can also interfere with communication between your brain, pituitary gland, and ovaries, creating a hormonal imbalance throughout your endocrine system. Furthermore, research shows that a diagnosis of infertility is as stressful for a woman as discovering she has HIV or cancer. How crazy is that? We're dealing with the Titanic here, folks. Acupuncture works to reverse the effects of stress by increasing circulation and regulating hormones.

MALE FACTOR INFERTILITY

Men who suffer from reduced sperm count and/or compromised sperm (the lack of sperm production) can benefit from acupuncture. Motility, morphology, and quantity can all benefit from acupuncture. By increasing blood flow and correcting underlying imbalances, acupuncture may remedy all of these after only a few months. It has also been proven to reduce the number of structural abnormalities in sperm.

MISCARRIAGE

There are numerous causes of miscarriage, including chromosomal abnormalities, illness, problems with the uterus or cervix, advanced maternal age, and hormonal imbalances. Acupuncture may help to prevent some causes of miscarriage by regulating hormones and optimizing progesterone production, which is essential to maintaining the uterus for a sustained pregnancy. It has been proven to help thicken the uterine lining and may protect against first-trimester miscarriages.

ANOVULATION

Research shows acupuncture and herbal medicine can induce ovulation in many patients experiencing anovulation.

Chapter 26
Buy One Get One Free (BOGO)

One of the hardest parts of IVF is the medication used during the stem cycle. It wreaks havoc on your mind and body. Thank God I don't have to do that again, lol. Totes to no stress. I get a couple of updates on the progress of the egg donor. Things are going superbly. What a relief! Thank God for her.

Egg retrieval day! Noah and I wait in the lobby, but I can tell the people at the desk are nervous, and they quickly usher us into a conference room. I know my Easter basket is somewhere in the vicinity. My mission becomes finding her. I excuse myself to go to the "bathroom" and start peeping in doors. I open one door, and I'm greeted by a nurse. "Are you trying to find the bathroom?" Caught. Crap.

"Oh, sorry. I'm just trying to find the conference room I was in." She redirects me. Mission failed. Noah shakes his head at me with a bitter smile. Any woman in my position would have done the same. Am I right, ladies?

An embryologist gets Noah for slap-happy fun time. He always loves me in the morning. He lethargically stands and mopes on the way to his X-rated fantasy hut.

Sarah calls, informing me they've received thirty-one mature eggs from the donor. I've only bought eight of them. She asks if I want to buy additional eggs before they fertilize. The idea is appealing, but at what cost? I have a little bit of sticker shock when Sarah casually informs me, "They are only $3,750 apiece." Yeah ... only ... I tell her I can't justify the cost. That's when she boosts that they'll give me a special: "Buy One, Get One Free." This is not a joke. I feel like I just transported into Walmart. Not even Target does BOGO. I still decline.

Now the fun numbers. Of the eight eggs, seven have fertilized, and six have made it to day 3 morulas. Dr. Jain says, though, that they are all still dividing. Again, thank God for twenty-year-olds.

Another three days pass, and three embryos make it to blastocyst. All excellent-looking, highly graded embryos. The doctor is unable to sync my cycle with the donor's, so we do a freeze on all of the embryos for a transfer in a few weeks.

My prep protocol for the frozen embryo transfer includes, yes, birth control, Lupron, estrogen, and progesterone. More medications, more medications, and more medications. Did I mention I have to take a few more medications? I've taken all of these before except Lupron, and holy headaches, I spent a good part of my Christmas break in Ohio, lying in a dark room with a cold compress on my head.

Noah accompanies me home for Christmas to avoid being alone for the holidays, since his mom has gone on a cruise. My family welcomes him with open arms.

At the start of my fertility journey, my niece, Ciara, began IUIs, and her second treatment was successful. She had a New Year's Eve 2016 baby. Her daughter, Makayla, has her first birthday party while we're still in Ohio. I have a hard time convincing myself I can make it through the party without crying.

She rents a room at the local VFW and hangs pink and purple decorations and helium balloons from the ceiling. The décor is bright, cheerful, and elegantly put together. My entire extended family brings presents and questions. *God help me. Deep breath. You can do this.* "When are you going to have a little one?" my Aunt Mimi chimes in. She always knows how to mind her own damn business. "That man you're with would have your babies. I see the way he looks at you. He's handsome. You know you're getting older and don't have much time. I mean, even your niece had to have some scientific help." *Jesus, it doesn't stop.*

"Will you excuse me? I should check on Noah."

I scurry off as fast as I can without running into another encounter. I plop down on a bench in the lobby and rest my head in my hands. "So, when are you going to have a baby?" Noah chuckles at his hideous joke.

"Shut up." I playfully push him away.

"You know, when I was your age, I already had three children and milked eighteen cows a day, plus took care of the whole house. What are you doing with your life?"

"Are you prepping me for my exam?"

"Why do you care what they think? You got out. You're living your dream. You're successful. You have great friends. You don't need them telling you what the norm is. The norm in LA is different. We do what we want. We don't want to live cookie-cutter lives.

"It's funny how you don't want to let your family know you're struggling. Like, they should be the ones you turn to. Instead, it's a bunch of one-uppers. Nah, let's go back in there and rock this joint!"

I can't help but force a smile. "Is that a smile I see? No, Lisa Hoover doesn't smile!" Noah pokes my face, helps me reluctantly stand, and bear-hugs the living shit out of me.

"Go get 'em, tiger!" He smacks my ass and shoos me back into the party.

My sister and niece place baby Makayla on the floor with the smash cake. Everyone gathers around, cheering and encouraging her to get messy. She doesn't get it. My niece walks over and sticks Makayla's hands in the cake. The hired photographer lies on the ground trying to get pictures of the momentous event. Once her hands are in the cake, it's no-holds-barred, and she destroys that poor, defenseless cake. Talk about a cake baby. Watching her, I imagine my own child going through this rite of passage. What I imagined would be a strenuous experience is essentially cathartic.

None of my family know I'm undergoing donor egg IVF. I don't want the pressure from everyone this time around. Being around youngsters makes me want to share what I am going through. I want a family. It isn't going to be standard, but it's going to happen in an alternative way. *I'm ready. I'm ready to be me, Lisa. You have to love me because you are my family. I don't need to be ashamed of what I'm doing.* I want to tell Noah my revelation. Where is Noah?

I round the corner and see him bouncing Makayla up and down in his arms. His beaming expression and glowing cheeks as he sways her side to side melt my lady parts. My stomach flutters, and my pulse races. *Why do you have to do this, Noah? I do not love you. I do not love you, but boy, you would make a great dad.* No, he's just my offspring's benefactor. He swings Makayla around in a circle, and she giggles. Noah catches me ogling them intently. I gracelessly grit my teeth and wave. Busted.

During this silent exchange, my sister asks, "What's going on between you and Noah?"

"I have no idea," I reply, semi-lying.

"There's something about him I can't put my finger on. Are you guys sleeping together?"

"Not exactly."

"What the hell does that mean?"

"I don't know, Suzanne," I proclaim.

"Be careful."

"Way past that."

"I know."

"Then why did you ask?"

"I don't want you to get hurt."

"Already happened. I don't have the distinguishing attributes he's looking for. He's picky."

"Whatever that means. Sounds stupid."

"I know, right? That's what *I* said!"

We continue to prepare dinner. Noah sits next to me and puts his arm on my chair, enjoying his stay and laughing at my dad's jokes. *Thanks for humoring my father, but not necessary.* My family grills Noah with questions about his life, and he takes them with ease. "I Can't Make You Love Me" (Bonnie Raitt, 1991) plays in my head over and over again. I have to stop questioning his affection. I know he cares for me. He loves me, but not in a romantic way, as he's made abundantly clear.

138

When I return to LA, I make a trip to The Psychic Eye Book Shop in Studio City. This place has renowned psychics who do readings throughout the day. Without providing any personal information other than my first name, I select the next available psychic, Allorah. The name itself sounds clairvoyant. What do I have to lose? I want her to tell me about Noah, the baby, and the future.

First off, she informs me that a Pisces and a Scorpio will have a baby (I'm a Scorpio and Noah is a Pisces—um, okay), but they are not a couple. "You, the Scorpio, are in love with the Pisces." (Duh, bitch.) "He doesn't feel the same way, but it's because he's scared." (Woah, wait! What?) I break down and tell her I am doing IVF treatments.

She says, "I see that, but you've been having sex to get pregnant. It's not been pleasurable. It's felt like a job. Your kids are laughing at you. I can't see if they are twins, but there are definitely two." She then tells me that they're waiting for us to get our shit together, submit to the truth, and get ready to be their parents.

"How do I do that?" I ask.

She replies, "You two need to stop playing games. You need to have fun again. You need to get drunk and have wild, passionate sex. Then the baby will come." That will never happen. Great. Dumb psychic. Waste of fifty bucks.

My transfer is two weeks away, and I need to let loose. My best friends and I decide to hit up a Hollywood club. I text Noah a quick invite, never expecting him to show up.

Shots! Shots! Shots!

Midway through our third round, Noah walks through the light across the dance floor. I'm drunk. Is this real?

This is not meant to be a night of debauchery. The stress of the past few months and the impending transfer seem to melt away with the sound of the music.

The bar has yet to close, but we're all tapped out. I'm thirty-eight—what do you expect? We each order our own Ubers. As I get in mine, Noah slides in next to me.

"I'm not driving to the Westside," I say, a bit tipsy.

"I know," he retorts. *Hold up! Is he coming home with me?*

I make us a drink and turn on the Weeknd mix on YouTube. He lies on my bed on his back. I'm on my stomach, talking. He leans down and kisses me. He never kissed me when we were trying to make a baby. He hasn't kissed me since the Tinder date. I think that's going to be it until he slowly moves his hands between my legs.

Oh my God*! The psychic! We're gonna have a baby!*

Chapter 27
The Celebrity Treatment

Leo agrees to chauffer me to acupuncture at 5:30 a.m. Dr. Alex doesn't usually come in that early, but he makes an exception because I'm in dire need.

We focus only on fertility points to nourish my uterus and increase blood flow. Rather than leaving me alone with music, he leads me in a guided meditation. He has me visualize the embryo entering my uterus, burrowing itself into the lining, and making a healthy home for nine months.

Leo also offers to drive me to the fertility clinic. We sit in traffic on the way to Santa Monica for the transfer. According to every single news source, LA has the world's worst traffic. It's *Office Space* on acid. It doesn't move. Most of the time, you're idle. I suggest books on tape. I'm glad I'm not driving so I can stay relaxed.

When I walk into the fertility clinic, the girls behind the counter are enthusiastic about the big day. They instantly ask, "Where's Noah?"

I lie. "Oh, he had an exam in class he couldn't get out of." The real reason: I didn't ask him to come. I thought it was too much pressure to put on him.

I'm led to a room I haven't seen before. It's reminiscent of my acupuncturist's office: crystal lamps, beautiful orchids, fluffy leather couches, and Zen music fill the room. This is already different from my last experience. The physician's assistant, Patty, a mid-forties brunette who's compassionate and kind, comes and tells me she's optimistic about this transfer. She's reviewed my charts, and she sees from my last ultrasound that my uterus has a triple stripe lining, whatever the hell that means. Sounds glorious. Basically, it's the perfect lining. She tells me that when transfers work, it's when there's a triple layer lining.

She's followed by a nurse, who brings me a Valium and a bottle of water. I'd prefer wine, but I understand. One thing I want to point out is they wanted my bladder only half full. Last time, I almost literally peed my pants, but this time, I'm relaxed and comfortable.

Dr. Jain hands me a picture of the blastocyst (which I carry in my wallet) and tells me the embryo we're transferring is a 4BA. It's excellent quality.

He eyes Leo inquisitively. I tell him, "Oh, it's fine. He's just my ex-boyfriend." I'm sure he's heard stranger things. I mean, we *are* in LA. He waves his hands in a "no judgement" sort of way.

Dr. Jain settles in at the foot of the table and swings a huge surgical lamp over my legs. Let there be light! I constantly wonder how the other doctor did it in the dark.

There is a sliding glass window between the embryologist lab and the transfer room. The embryologist hands Dr. Jain a vial with my name on it, and it's triple-checked by the nurse and the physician's assistant.

The embryologist prepares the catheter with my little baby. Patty does an abdominal ultrasound while Dr. Jain guides the catheter into my uterus. He is exceptionally gentle. I don't feel a thing. A small white speck in my uterus appears on the ultrasound. My baby is home! This is a huge deal. *Huge.*

Patty prints a picture of my uterus with the white speck. When she hands me the picture, she exclaims that I should frame it. "Most people can't say they have an image of the moment their life changed!"

This procedure is followed by another visit to Dr. Alex. He does acupuncture and moxa treatments on several parts of my body. It's only 11:00 a.m., and I've already had quite the morning.

On my way home, I insist we go to the McDonald's drive-thru. I have to order French fries. I've seen Facebook posts with pictures of women holding McDonald's fries right after an IVF transfer. It may be a wives' tale, but people claim it helps implantation. It may sound crazy, but I have yet to attempt it, and I'm willing to try anything and everything.

For the last transfer, I drank pomegranate juice and cut up pineapple with the core to eat over five days, as the core contains bromelain. Bromelain reduces inflammation, thins blood, and is believed to aid in implantation. Since it didn't work last time, I'm not doing it again. No one will convince me otherwise

This time I declare I will not symptom spot, journal, or take any home pregnancy tests. To avoid temptation, I don't buy any, and I make sure to use up the ones I already have on my dog. I'm kidding. Can you imagine? I bet you can—you're almost done with this book.

I'm grateful Dr. Jain tests one week after transfer instead of the usual two. I can handle a one-week wait, I think. I'm not sure yet. I feel like I can. Maybe ask me in a few days?

Although I'm not looking for symptoms, it's hard to deny the mild cramps and pinpricks in my uterus. About five days into the wait, I experience chest pain—the internal kind, pulling, stretching, aching. Wait—the only other time I noticed this was during my chemical pregnancy. Could this possibly have worked? I repeat the mantra "Happy, Healthy, Pregnant."

Chapter 28
Say What?

To avoid an hour-long trip in traffic for a blood draw, I get a prescription and head to my local LabCorp. On the way, I pass a Burger King, and boy, am I hungry, so I get a Croissan'wich with egg, ham, and cheese. I arrive just before nine and am taken to the back to see a phlebotomist named Patty. It's a sign: Dr. Jain's physician's assistant is named Patty. There are no coincidences in life, according to Deepak Chopra. She's a Chatty Cathy and my personal cheerleader. My bloodwork is ordered STAT, and it will take no longer than four hours for Dr. Jain to get the results.

I meet Leo for lunch, anticipating the results. We opt to play a fun game of search-and-seek. While we sit on the outdoor patio, Leo uploads one of my baby mama's profile pictures to Google Reverse Image Search. We're instantly greeted by a plethora of provocative portraits. Turns out she's an Instagram underwear model. I immediately follow her. She has fifty thousand followers. She won't notice one more, unless she buys her followers' names. Then I might be screwed.

I discover the unedited version of her donor profile pic, ass cheeks and all. I mean, she is all about her butt. I'm relieved she looks better without fake lips. I'm happy I found her Insta and realize she no longer looks fake Hollywood or like a duck. One thing's for sure: if I have a daughter, she will *not* be following in these footsteps. After all, morals are learned, right?

My phone buzzes. It's the clinic. My hands tremble as I attempt to answer it. I'm greeted by Patty. As she talks, I'm not hearing her speech but analyzing her tone. She seems upbeat. This has to be good, right? "I just got your results," she declares. "It's positive!" Tears roll down my face, and Leo consoles me.

I blurt out, "It worked!" Leo stops rubbing my back and decides "Why not record Lisa while she is hysterically crying?" I don't know whether to punch or kiss him. I'm informed we will do a repeat blood test in two days.

I call my mom, and she answers nervously. She hears the quiver in my voice, and I can sense a letdown. "You're going to be a grandma again."

She snivels in exultation. This situation has been arduous on us all.

For the second beta test, because I'm superstitious, I decide to repeat the exact steps as the day of my first beta. I stop at Burger King, I arrive before nine, and I request Patty.

I don't even know Patty the phlebotomist, and she gives me a hug because it worked. Let the four-hour wait begin again. Or the 4HW, as I like to call it. I think I'm pretty fancy. Although I was excited by the positive news two days ago, I've been through this before, only to be disappointed when the beta number dropped rather than rose. Because of this emotional roller coaster, you want to be optimistic, but you also don't want to care.

The clinic calls sooner than they did with the first beta. Patty jumps right in: "Numbers look great. You're pregnant!" They request one final beta a week later.

I slide down my kitchen cabinet, barely feeling my hands to dial anyone's number. I bask in joy. What do I do next? Well, I'll tell you: I dance and chant, *"I'm pregnant! I'm pregnant! I'm pregnant!"* This only lasts a few minutes because I run out of breath. I can't stop smiling, beaming ear to ear so wide my mouth hurts. I don't care. You know why? Because *I'm fucking pregnant*! Hey, guess what? Did I mention I'm pregnant? Like for real, for real. One hundred percent pregnant.

Third beta day arrives, and like Groundhog Day, I repeat the same steps, my good luck charm. Since I've already committed to a bachelorette party, I jump in a car with my girlfriends and head to Vegas. On the road, I receive another phone call from Patty—shocker—who informs me my hCG numbers are higher than expected. Things are looking good, and I schedule my first ultrasound for a week later.

The girls ask me what the call was about. I lie and explain it was my doctor's office rescheduling an appointment. They ask why I'm beaming, and again, with my amazing lying skills, I proclaim, "I'm excited about this girls' trip!" Now I'm thinking, *Fuck! How am I going to hide my not drinking?*

We rent a suite and see the Backstreet Boys that night. You know, the usual. I pour beer out of a can and replace it with apple juice. The bartender serves me shots of water, pretending it's vodka. I can hide the drinking, but I can't hide my fatigue. I'm having a hard time keeping up.

A week flies by, and I'm technically six weeks and one day pregnant. Entering the clinic, I'm welcomed with embraces and congratulations from the front desk girls and Sarah. I remind Sarah of what she told me three months ago about how my journey would end here. Those words replayed in my head and kept me going.

Dr. Jain meets me in an ultrasound room. He goes to shake my hand, but I hug him instead and profess my gratitude. Endeared, he says he's happy he could help. He makes a request: "One more thing, Lisa. Will you bring the baby in after it's born? So many people say they will, and they never do."

"I will. I promise."

As he commences the ultrasound, I can tell from the smile on his face that everything looks good. He points to the tiny white flicker on the screen and explains that it's the heart beating nice and strong. The baby is measuring on time and looks great.

The doctor is going to keep me on progesterone and estrogen for the first twelve weeks to help sustain the pregnancy. They play key roles in preparing for pregnancy. Any drop in the level of progesterone can impact the health of the uterine lining, which in turn can lead to spotting, bleeding, and, ultimately, a miscarriage.

Fun fact: Most doctors say not to have sex until after you hear the heartbeat. It's not really sex that's the concern; it's the female orgasm. Avoid a contracting uterus with a newly implanted baby. I will abstain the whole first trimester.

Chapter 29
Is This Normal?

Ecstatic, I head over to Noah's after the ultrasound. I'm bouncing foot to foot and beaming ear to ear, excited to show him the beautiful picture of my baby. Yes, I said *my* baby! I knock on the door, and to my surprise, a skank answers, wearing Noah's favorite baseball tee. It's obvious they've had a sleepover. I've always known he has his own life, but it's been sheltered from me. Now, seeing it in the flesh, I'm completely devastated.

Noah slides to the door nonchalantly. "Oh, hey. How have you been?" I glare deep into his light blue eyes, holding back the waterworks. I don't want him to see me cry. I jab the ultrasound picture into his chest and sprint to my car. I will blame my outburst on the hormones and, possibly, the pregnancy.

I remain in my car for a moment, bawling, dry heaving, and pounding my steering wheel. *What does he see in her? Why her? She looks like he picked her up at Pico and Sepulveda. What is she? His drug dealer? I guess she is pretty, in a heroine-chic, haven't-eaten-in-weeks, androgynous sort of way. I don't understand. Are these the fucking attributes he's looking for?*

I clutch my gut. Tight convulsions pulse in my lower abdomen. Wincing in agony, I tell myself to calm down. *Breathe in. Breathe out. Stop this.* I muster up the strength to start my car and drive home.

I stagger to the bathroom and wipe. Instinctively, I always look at the toilet paper. As a woman going through fertility treatments, you always check the TP to make sure. It's clear. I wipe again and do a double take. Is that pink? Is it pink? Oh my God! The blood drains from my face. I'm feeling sick to my stomach. *I can't lose this baby. I can't lose this baby over stressing about a dense dimwit I have no future with.* The nurse had told me spotting can be normal but that if it got worse, like a period, to let her know.

I wake up the next morning, and the twinge pink has turned to red. It's the weekend, so I have no choice but to rush to the ER.

I'm given a nurse that does OB stuff, and she lets me know that spotting doesn't always indicate a miscarriage. She says there could be several reasons, but she's not giving me definitive answers. *Why won't anybody just give me an answer? Stop peddling around the subject. I'm a big girl.*

The head doctor decides to do bloodwork, check my hCG levels, and do an ultrasound. During the ultrasound, I draw a deep breath through my nose when I saw the baby's heartbeat. Relief fills my entire body. The baby is measuring on time and has a strong heartbeat of 150. Lower heart rates are supposed to be boys, and higher ones mean girls—not an exact science. This heartbeat indicates a girl. I'm filled with anticipation and delight, but I try not to get my hopes up.

I have a negative blood type, and because Noah's and the egg donor's are positive, they give me a RhoGAM shot. Typically, you don't get this shot until week twenty-eight, but because I'm bleeding, they administer it early. My hCG levels are 97,000, well above normal. Although they can't rule out a miscarriage, they tell me everything is fine. They tell me I have to relax, take it easy, and not lift anything heavy. Don't have to ask me twice!

I realize how attached I already am to this pregnancy. Two days later, the pink is gone. The storm has passed, and I can finally let my hair down.

POSSIBLE REASONS YOU CAN SPOT

-   Twenty percent of women have bleeding during pregnancy, especially in the first trimester
-   Implantation bleeding
-   Sexual intercourse
-   Gynecological exam
-   Heavy lifting
-   Heavy exercise
-   Subchorionic hemorrhage
-   A small percentage of women do bleed during their entire pregnancy. Many mistake it for a period, which is how we ended up with the show *I Didn't Know I Was Pregnant.*

Chapter 30
Graduation

Haven't communicated with Noah in a couple of weeks. It's getting easier. I am extra ecstatic because it's graduation day! I've moved past the reproductive endocrinologist and back to a regular OB/GYN at "University" hospital. Don't worry; it's a different doctor. This one I like. I've seen him for years for annual checkups.

I'm one of the cool kids. I sit in the waiting area among other women with bumps. I'm developing a baby and no longer trying. My mission is complete.

The peanut no longer looks like a blob with a heartbeat. It's taken on human form. It's wiggling about, kicking and stretching. Once they do the audio of the heartbeat, it hits me. *This is happening. There is a human growing inside my midriff.* The doctor prints the most glorious picture I have ever gotten to encounter.

We sit in his office and make a calendar of milestones and appointments. All the scans and dates put into perspective how complete my life is at this moment. We discuss having a planned C-section for two reasons. First, the hardware in my back from previous surgeries will prevent the anesthesiologist from being able to administer an epidural. When I got my HSG and my uterus contracted, it was the worst fucking pain I had ever felt, and I have experienced my fair share of pain, so I know I'm not a candidate for natural childbirth. Secondly, natural labor can reinjure the vertebra in my lower back.

The doctor and I discuss doing a noninvasive prenatal test (NIPT). I agree because we didn't do PGD/PGS testing on the donor egg embryo. An NIPT reveals your baby's risk for genetic disorders and chromosomal abnormalities. It also reveals the gender, which is really why I want this done. I always like to open Christmas presents early.

I'm in the lab, and they keep filling more vials. How many are they going to take? I don't usually have a problem getting my blood drawn, but I might have found my limit. He tests for everything you could possibly test for. When I get the results, at least I know all my organs and bodily functions are operating correctly. The NIPT we do is through Panorama. The results could take up to ten days. Is this going to be another two-week wait situation? Am I going to be checking their website every day? Affirmative.

Eight days later, the website shows that the doctor has the results! I call, and I have to leave a voicemail. Unacceptable. That night, I visualize my life with a boy or a girl. I don't care. A life with a girl will be dress-up, doing nails, dance class, and girl talk. A life with a boy will be monster trucks, sports—damn, I need to research what you do with boys.

I get the call first thing in the morning and hear "Congratulations! It's a girl!" My heart sinks. More importantly, she is at low risk for any genetic or chromosomal abnormalities. Now off to Target—I need girl clothes!

Chapter 31
Honesty is the Best Policy

From the beginning, I knew I was going to be honest with my child. Psychologists say that is the best thing to do. I want my child to know I wanted her badly, unconditionally. Hiding her origins makes it seem secretive and/or shameful. I want her to know it took the gifts of a few special people to make our family complete. I'm not embarrassed by using donors, and I don't feel "less than" because my child doesn't have my genetics. She is my child, plain and simple. While I am open with close friends and family, I don't publicly broadcast her origins. I'll let her decide who she wants to tell.

I thought I might be sad to not have a genetically related child, but I rarely think about it. What's most important to me is being the best mom I can be to this exquisitely charming girl. I am beyond grateful to Noah and the egg donor for their generosity and providing what I was missing to produce my family.

FACEBOOK PAGES FOR DONOR FAMILIES

Donor Conceived Offspring, Siblings, Parents
Donor Conception Support Group
Egg Donor Angels Parents of Donor Conceived Children Support Group

CHILDREN'S BOOKS FOR
UNCONVENTIONAL FAMILIES

Hope and Will Have a Baby by Irene Celcer. Ages 5–8. This series of books focuses on surrogacy, egg donation, embryo donation, sperm donation, and adoption. The beginning and end of each book are the same, but the middle sections are specific to each topic. Contains some religious overtones.

How Babies and Families Are Made: There Is More Than One Way! by Patricia Schaffer. Ages 5–9. Surveys the different ways in which children are conceived, developed, born, and become parts of families, examining special situations such as artificial insemination, caesarean births, and families with adopted children or stepchildren.

Just the Baby for Me by Barbara Sue Levin. Ages 5–9. Story of a single mother who has a child using donor sperm.

The Donor Conception Network has a series of books called *Our Story* that discuss the use of donor sperm. *My Story* covers donor sperm for a heterosexual couple, while two books entitled *Our Story* cover sperm donation for single mothers and lesbian couples. www.dcnetwork.org

Before You Were Born by Janice Grimes, RN. A series of books on sperm donation. Ages 3–5.

A Baby for Mummy: Explaining Artificial Insemination for Young Children by Julie Cavaney. Ages 0–8 years old. Introduces the concept of a sperm donor through artificial insemination to children born from sperm donors to single mothers. This book celebrates how much our children are wanted and loved.

God's Magical Dust by Karolina Dembinska-Lemus. Ages 5–8. A bilingual children's book about the role of God in third-party reproduction. First half is the English version; second half is the Spanish version. Includes relevant Bible quotes.

Wish by Matthew Cordell. Ages 3–5. When an elephant couple decides it is time to have a child, unexpected challenges arise but, at last, the pair's deepest wish comes true.

Your Story: IVF by Kylie and Matthew Hill. Ages 5–8. A children's book that explains the standard IVF process to assist baby making.

The Pea That Was Me: An IVF Story by Kimberly Kluger-Bell. Ages 3–5. Reading this charming storybook to your preschooler is a wonderful way to introduce them to the fact you wanted them very much but had trouble having them. The very basic fact it takes an egg and a sperm to make a baby is introduced.

Families Come in Many Forms by Bella Mei Wong. Along the way, Alex meets his friends' families—traditional, adopted, divorced, blended, IVF, same-sex, and others. These families are not presented as "different" but are treated as a normal part of today's world.

My Little Dish by Sari Dennis. For every parent who has experienced the emotional roller coaster called infertility, this book has been written to provide you with a point at which you may begin to discuss your child's conception.

The Dancing Fish and the Clever Crab by Ms. Reen. Ages 2–10. This book was written as an aid to parents who conceived a child via the use of donor eggs or sperm. The decision whether to disclose the child's genetic origins to him or her is an important one for parents.

The Extra Button by Jules Blundell. Benny and Rose wanted more than anything to have their own family. In this gorgeous picture book, Jules uses a story about a gingerbread couple as a metaphor to explain the difficult concept of donor conception to young children.

It Takes Love (and some other stuff) to Make a Baby by L. L. Bird. The book introduces children to several concepts and vocabulary words such as "ovaries," "uterus," "pregnant," "sperm," "egg," "testicles," "sperm donor," and "sperm bank" and explains what each term means when it comes up in the context of the description of how babies are made in two-mom families.

God Wanted Me! God Created Me! by Teresa Adams. Ages 5–8 years old. This book takes a deeply religious approach with a child conceived via sperm or egg donation. The book aims to comfort the child who may feel unsettled by the fact that they do not know their biological parent.

Megan and Mommy by Elizabeth Reed. A story of being a single mother who chooses to go to a clinic and use a sperm donor to have a child.

Mom, Mama and Me ... and How I Came to Be! by Tina Rella. Ages 3–5. This book takes a family-building approach and employs the "families are made differently" and a little bit of "the helper" scripts. Full-color illustrations depict a multiracial lesbian couple.

Mommy, Did I Grow in Your Tummy? by Elaine R. Gordon, PhD. Ages 3–8. The book explains five different methods for having a baby: sperm donation, egg donation, surrogacy, in vitro fertilization, and adoption. These methods, all introduced with the proper vocabulary, are all explained in a way that a child could understand them.

Family Stew: Two Moms Use a Sperm Donor to Build their Family by Linda Stamm. Ages 7+. This vividly illustrated and humorous children's book is a wonderful way for children conceived via donor sperm to learn about their origin.

Chapter 32
Modern Family

What is this, the twenty-first century? Family units don't all consist of a mom and a dad. There are two moms, two dads, single dads, single moms, siblings raising siblings, adopted families, foster families, and everything in between. A family is built on love, not social standards. I may be a single mom, but my enchanted daughter will have strong male influences to guide, love, and support her.

Leo has been there for me since I was a teen. He protects me like a parent. He has already guaranteed me that he'll be even more protective over this baby girl, and she won't date until she's thirty. Fine by me!

Noah and I have lunch in the Palisades. I approach his table on the sidewalk patio area, and there, in plain sight, is the ultrasound picture. He begins the conversation by apologizing to me about the whore. "But you know that will never be you." A dampness comes over my eyes. "Yes, I do love you, but I am not in love with you. I just don't have those type of feelings."

A tear falls from my face. This is tough to hear, although I've known for months. He has been distant because seeing the ultrasound makes this whole experience real now. He has to do some soul searching to detach himself as her parent and accept he's only the donor.

"Well, how do you see this playing out?" I ask, my voice quivering.

"I was thinking maybe an uncle figure. I want to be in their life, but I don't want them to know I'm their dad, as I fear they will resent me for not being in their life full time."

Have I been living in a fantasy of happily ever after with Noah? I inhale deeply and comprehend that it's always been about the baby and not about Noah.

"It's a little girl."

Noah smiles. "Wow, she's going to be a really pretty girl. I want to teach her to play guitar."

I thank him for standing by my side, never giving up, and being a source of love and support. This is way more than he ever signed up for, yet here he is, chatting about ways to be in the baby's life. Little did I know that swiping right three years ago would result in my perfect DNA. What was meant to be a one-night stand has turned into a forever friendship.

There's a lot more discussion to be had about Noah's role and sharing his identity with this girl. I plan on seeking the advice of a psychologist/psychiatrist who specializes in donor-conceived children. I want to do what's best for my daughter.

"In my daughter's eyes, I am a hero. I am strong and wise. And I know no fear. But the truth is plain to see, she was sent to rescue me" (Martina McBride, 2003).

Chapter 33
To My Future Child

Bardot,

I lie here writing this letter while you are tucked safely inside my womb, growing strong. I've loved you from the moment I was told I was pregnant. You've stolen my heart. I count the days until we meet, and I embrace you in my arms. I dream of you—your smile, the twinkle in your eyes, your heart beating against my chest.

All children are blessings. You are not only a blessing but a miracle. Mommy has wanted you for so very long. Thirty-eight years, to be exact. I've hoped, wished, and prayed for you. I'm incredibly lucky you selected me to be your mom. I've fought for you, cried for you, and loved for you. It took special people coming together to allow you to join this world. Everyone is overjoyed for you and grateful you are growing strong. You are healthy and already undeniably beautiful. At my doctor's appointment today, I got to see you. I love watching you wiggle and stretch your arms and legs. You've become quite the acrobat. I rub my tummy often. I hope you can feel I'm here, saying hello, and I will always be around whenever you need me.

I often think about our future together. The cuddles, the love, the kisses. You growing into a smart and clever girl. I picture trips to the beach, strolls in the park, blowing bubbles, pushing you on a swing, swimming lessons, and play time with others we know.

My fur babies (Johnny and Fred) are eager to meet you as well. They lie on my stomach and lick me playfully, knowing you are with us. They pay extra close attention to you moving in my belly. They will be the best brothers ever to you! They will guard you and give you endless kisses.

Your grandma, grandpa, aunts, uncles, and cousins are thrilled you are joining our family. They know how long I've dreamt of you. They have been supportive and encouraging of this journey to bring you home.

I'm especially excited for you to meet Leo. He is our family. He never gave up on my dream to conceive you, and he has been there every step of the way. He loves hearing all about you and seeing your pictures. He will be in the room the day you are born. He already loves you and will protect you with his life. You can always count on him. For anything! We are both lucky to have him in our lives. Feels like a lifetime. He cares for me and will care for you. He's an angel sent from above.

I visualize our relationship throughout the years—girl talks, dance classes, you becoming valedictorian. No pressure. I've had a great life, but I want yours to surpass mine. Having you has proved to me you really can achieve anything your heart desires. There is no limit to what you can achieve.

Your story may be different from others, but that is what makes you special.

I'll be your strength when you are feeling weak. I will be your shelter when you have nowhere else to go. I will be your light when you are feeling down. I will be your support when you need help. I will be there for you no matter what the circumstances, no matter the sticky situations and the tough decisions. Always remember I will be there. When we fight, if there is a storm, after your first breakup, I will be your shoulder to cry on. I will be there.

Unconditionally Loved,
Mom

Glossary

2WW: Two-week wait. The estimated period of time between a pregnancy attempt and the date when it is most likely a pregnancy test is able to accurately indicate if the attempt was successful or not.

ABORTION: The deliberate termination of a human pregnancy.

AC: Assisted conception. A pregnancy resulting from any intervening medical technology that completely or partially replaces sexual intercourse as means of conception.

AF: Aunt Flow. Period or menstruation.

ALP: Alkaline phosphatase. An enzyme that liberates phosphate under alkaline conditions and is made in the liver, bones, and other tissues. Abnormally high serum levels may indicate bone disease, liver disease, or bile duct obstruction.

AMH: Anti-Müllerian hormone. A substance produced by granulosa cells in ovarian follicles. It is first made in primary follicles that advance from the primordial follicle stage. At these stages, follicles are microscopic and cannot be seen by ultrasound. AMH levels mean egg quantity.

AMPULLA: The third portion of the fallopian tube. It is an intermediate dilated portion that curves over the ovary. It is the most common site of human fertilization. The word "ampulla" is from the Latin word for flask.

ANEUPLOIDY: The presence of an abnormal number of chromosomes in a cell; for example, a human cell having forty-five or forty-seven chromosomes instead of the usual forty-six. An extra or missing chromosome is a common cause of genetic disorders, including some birth defects. Some cancer cells also have abnormal numbers of chromosomes.

ANTICOAGULANT: The process of hindering the clotting of blood. Helps increase blood flow to the uterus, nourishing the lining.

ANTRAL FOLLICLES: A measure of egg supply for the future (ovarian reserve); helps predict chances of a successful IVF. A fairly simple test to perform with high-quality ultrasound equipment.

ANUS: The opening at the end of the alimentary canal through which solid waste matter leaves the body. True definition.

AO: Anovulatory. No ovulation occurred.

AREOLA: A small circular area, in particular the ring of pigmented skin surrounding the nipple.

ART: Assisted reproductive technology. Technology used to achieve pregnancy with procedures such as fertility medication, in vitro fertilization, and surrogacy. Used primarily for infertility treatments.

ASA: Anti-sperm antibody. Proteins in blood, vaginal fluids, or semen that damage or kill sperm.

ARTIFICIAL INSEMINATION: See IUI.

ATP: Adenosine triphosphate. The energy currency of life. A high-energy molecule found in every cell. Its job is to store and supply the cell with needed energy.

BBT: Basal body temperature. The lowest body temperature reached during rest or sleep.

BCP: Birth control pills. Oral contraceptives for women containing the hormones estrogen and progesterone or progesterone alone, which inhibit ovulation, fertilization, or implantation of a fertilized ovum, causing temporary infertility.

BD: Baby dance. A playful way to describe sex.

BETA: hCG pregnancy test. A blood test to assess the level of beta hCG in the blood, an accurate way of assessing for pregnancy.

BFN: Big fat negative. A negative pregnancy test outcome. Not to be confused with Big Fucking No, but basically the same thing.

BFP: Big fat positive. A positive pregnancy test outcome.

BLASTOCYST: A thin-walled hollow structure in early embryonic development containing a cluster of cells called the inner cell mass (ICM) from which the embryo arises.

BLASTOMERES: A cell formed by cleavage of a fertilized ovum.

BMS: Baby-making sex.

BROMELAIN: An enzyme extract derived from the stems of pineapples, although it exists in all parts of the fresh plant and fruit. The extract has a history of folk medicine use.

BW: Blood work.

C#: Cycle number.

CD: Cycle day. Which day you're up to in your menstrual cycle.

CGH: Comparative genomic hybridization. A DNA diagnostic technique that compares an embryo's chromosomes with a standard set to check for chromosome abnormalities.

CHEMICAL PREGNANCY: A conception that has measurable hCG but does not develop far enough to be seen on an ultrasound. Unsuccessful, and the only evidence an early pregnancy existed is the measurement of hCG in a woman's blood or urine.

CLOMID: A medication used to jumpstart ovulation. Also known as CloMAD because of its side effects.

CM: Cervical mucus (also known as cervical fluid). It is fluid produced by your cervix due to increased estrogen as you approach ovulation.

CONCEPTION: Become pregnant with a child.

CORPUS LUTEUM: A hormone-secreting structure that develops in an ovary after an ovum has been discharged but degenerates after a few days unless pregnancy has begun.

CP: Cervical position. A secondary optional fertility sign. The cervix changes throughout the menstrual cycle in response to the hormone estrogen. During nonfertile times, the cervix is closed, firm, and low.

CRYOBANK: A facility or enterprise that collects and stores human sperm from sperm donors for use by people who need donor-provided sperm to achieve pregnancy.

CS: Caesarean section. A surgical operation for delivering a child by cutting through the wall of the mother's abdomen.

CUMULUS CELLS: A cluster of cells that surround the oocyte, both in the ovarian follicle and after ovulation.

CVS: Chorionic villi sampling. A test during pregnancy that checks the baby for some genetic abnormalities such as Down syndrome.

DD: Dear Daughter.

DE: Donor egg. Egg donation is the process by which a fertile woman provides one or several eggs (also known as ova or oocytes) to infertile recipients for purposes of assisted reproduction. After the eggs have been retrieved from the donor, the role of the egg donor is complete.

DNA: Deoxyribonucleic acid. A self-replicating material present in nearly all living organisms as the main constituent of chromosomes. It is the carrier of genetic information.

DONOR EMBRYOS: Embryos are donated by couples undergoing IVF who become pregnant and no longer need unused fertilized eggs. The donated embryo is then transferred into the recipient.

DH: Dear Husband.

DP: Dear Partner.

DPO: Days post-ovulation. Usually about fifteen days past ovulation is when your period starts.

DPR: Days post-retrieval. Refers to the number of days that have passed since the embryo transfer portion of an in vitro fertilization (IVF) procedure. Several significant milestones that occur after an embryo has been transferred to a uterus are measured in days post-transfer (DPT), including implantation, embryo development, and testing for pregnancy.

DPT: Days post-transfer. A term used to count the days that have passed since an embryo was transferred to a uterus during an in vitro fertilization procedure.

DS: Dear Son.

DS: Donor sperm. A donation by a male of his sperm, principally for the purpose of insemination of a female who is not his sexual partner. Sperm may be donated privately and directly to the intended recipient or through a sperm bank or fertility clinic.

ED: Egg donor. See DE (Donor Egg).

EDD: Estimated due date. Term describing the estimated delivery date for a pregnant woman. Normal pregnancies last between 37–42 weeks.

EGG QUALITY: The presence of genetically normal or abnormal eggs. Varies largely with a woman's reproductive age. With advanced age, the risk for chromosomal (genetic) abnormalities increases, and the egg quality becomes poor.

EGG RETRIEVAL: Transvaginal oocyte retrieval (TVOR), also referred to as oocyte retrieval (OCR), is a technique used in IVF to remove oocytes from the ovary of a woman, enabling fertilization outside the body.

EJACULATION: The action of ejecting semen from the body.

EMBRYO: An unborn or unhatched offspring in the process of development, in particular a human offspring during the period from the second to eighth week after fertilization (after which it is usually termed a fetus).

EMBRYO GRADING: One of the most subjective things an embryologist does in an IVF lab. Embryologists will make their choice of which embryos to transfer or cryopreserve based upon a grade given to the embryos. All embryo gradings are subjective. Refers to how the cells in the embryos look.

EMBRYO IMPLANTATION: A process in which a developing embryo, moving as a blastocyst through a uterus, makes contact with the uterine wall and remains attached to it until birth.

ENDO: Endometriosis. A condition resulting from the appearance of endometrial tissue outside the uterus, causing pelvic pain. Has been linked to infertility.

ENDO: Endometrium. The mucous membrane lining of the uterus, which thickens during the menstrual cycle in preparation for possible implantation of an embryo.

ENDOCRINE SYSTEM: The collection of glands producing hormones that regulate metabolism, growth and development, tissue function, sexual function, reproduction, sleep, and mood, among other things.

EPIDIDYMIS: A coiled segment of the spermatic ducts that stores spermatozoa while they mature and then transports the spermatozoa between the testis and the tube connecting the testes with the urethra (vas deferens).

EPIGENETICS: The study of changes in organisms caused by modification of gene expression rather than alteration of the genetic code itself.

EPO: Evening primrose oil. An oil extracted from the seeds of the evening primrose plant. It contains gamma-linolenic acid and is used in complementary and alternative medicine, especially in the treatment of premenstrual syndrome.

EPT: Early pregnancy test. A test for pregnancy that can give the quickest result after fertilization is a rosette inhibition assay for early pregnancy factor (EPF). Most chemical tests for pregnancy look for the presence of the beta subunit of human chorionic gonadotropin (hCG) in the blood or urine.

EPU: Egg pick-up. Procedure to collect eggs from the ovaries; also called ovum pick-up (OPU).

ERA: Endometrial receptivity analysis.

ERECTION: An enlarged and rigid state of the penis, typically during sexual excitement.

ESTROGEN: Any of a group of steroid hormones that promote the development and maintenance of female characteristics of the body.

ET: Embryo transfer. Refers to a step in the process of assisted reproduction in which embryos are placed into the uterus of a female with the intent to establish pregnancy.

EUPLOID: The normal number of chromosomes for a species.

EWCM: Egg white cervical mucus. Fertile cervical mucus.

FA: Freeze all. The developing embryos are frozen by a process called vitrification and stored until they are transferred at a later time.

FALLOPIAN TUBE: A pair of tubes along which eggs travel from the ovaries to the uterus.

FERTILITY DRUGS: Drugs that enhance reproductive fertility. For women, fertility medication is used to stimulate follicle development of the ovary.

FERTILIZED EGG: The union of a human egg and sperm, usually occurring in the ampulla of the fallopian tube. The result of this union is the production of a zygote cell, or fertilized egg, initiating prenatal development.

FET: Frozen embryo transfer. A cycle in which a frozen embryo from a previous fresh IVF cycle is thawed and transferred back into a woman's uterus. This means you won't have to undergo another cycle of hormone stimulation and egg collection.

FET: Fresh embryo transfer. Follows your IVF cycle of ovarian stimulation and happens very soon after your initial egg retrieval procedure. Transfer can occur one to six days after successful fertilization. These days, most clinics allow the embryo to reach the blastocyst stage before transferring. This is usually on day 5 or 6.

FF: Fertility friend.

166

FMU: First morning urine. A sample of urine is expelled immediately after waking up and is recommended for use with most home pregnancy tests.

FOLLICLE: A fluid-filled sac containing an immature egg.

FP: Follicular phase. The part of the monthly cycle before ovulation.

FRER: First Response Early Result™. Early pregnancy test.

FS: Frozen sperm. Method of preserving semen for future artificial insemination.

FS: Fertility specialist. Assists couples and sometimes individuals who want to become parents but for medical reasons have been unable to achieve this goal via the natural course.

FSA: Fertility Society of Australia. One in six couples in Australia and New Zealand suffer infertility.

FSBU: Frozen sperm backup. For some odd reason, the man can't perform the day of fertilization or there is a decrease in sperm count. So, abstain from ejaculating forty-eight hours before.

FSH: Follicle-stimulating hormone. Helps control the menstrual cycle and production of eggs by the ovaries.

GENETIC LINK: The tendency of DNA sequences that are close together on a chromosome to be inherited together during the meiosis phase of sexual reproduction.

GENETIC TESTING: A medical test that identifies changes in chromosomes, genes, or proteins. The results of a genetic test can confirm or rule out a suspected genetic condition or help determine a person's chance of developing or passing on a genetic disorder.

GIFT: Gamete intrafallopian transfer. Eggs from the woman are collected, mixed with sperm from the man in a petri dish, and then placed directly inside the fallopian tubes, where fertilization can occur.

GNH: Gonadotropin-releasing hormone. A hormone secreted by the hypothalamus that stimulates the anterior lobe of the pituitary gland to release gonadotropins (such as luteinizing hormone and follicle-stimulating hormone).

HCG: Human chorionic gonadotropin. Hormone detected by pregnancy tests.

HGH: Human growth hormone. A peptide hormone that stimulates growth, cell reproduction, and cell regeneration in humans and other animals. It is thus very important in human development.

HPT: Home pregnancy test.

HSG: Hysterosalpingogram. Special kind of X-ray of your uterus and fallopian tubes to evaluate female fertility. A dye is injected through the cervix into the uterus and fallopian tubes.

HYPOTHALAMUS: Controls the autonomic nervous system and the secretion of hormones by the pituitary gland. Through these nerve and hormone channels, the hypothalamus regulates many vital biological processes, including body temperature, blood pressure, thirst, hunger, and the sleep-wake cycle.

HYSTEROSCOPY: The inspection of the uterine cavity by endoscopy with access through the cervix. It allows for the diagnosis of intrauterine pathology and serves as a method for surgical intervention.

IC: Internet cheapie(s). A pregnancy test.

IC: Incompetent cervix (also called cervical insufficiency). A condition that occurs when weak cervical tissue contributes to premature birth or the loss of an otherwise healthy pregnancy. If you have an incompetent cervix, your cervix might begin to open too soon, causing you to give birth too early.

IC: Intercourse. Physical sexual contact between individuals involving the genitalia of at least one person.

ICM: Inner cell mass. Mass of cells inside the primordial embryo that, once fertilized, will eventually give rise to the definitive structure of the fetus.

ICSI: Intracytoplasmic sperm injection. Injection by a microneedle of a single sperm into an egg that has been obtained from an ovary; followed by transfer of the egg to an incubator, where fertilization takes place, and then by introduction of the fertilized egg into a female's uterus.

IMSI: Intracytoplasmic morphologically selected sperm injection. Represents a more sophisticated way of ICSI whereby, prior to injection, the spermatozoon is selected at a high magnification.

INFERTILITY: Inability to conceive children. Some definitions say this is a disease of the reproductive system defined by the failure to achieve a clinical pregnancy after twelve or more months of regular unprotected sexual intercourse.

INSEMINATION: The introduction of semen into a woman or a female animal by natural or artificial means.

INTRAUTERINE: Within the uterus.

IUI: Intrauterine insemination. A fertility treatment that involves placing sperm inside a woman's uterus to facilitate fertilization. The goal of IUI is to increase the number of sperm reaching the fallopian tubes and subsequently increase the chance of fertilization.

IVF: In vitro fertilization. A medical procedure whereby an egg is fertilized by sperm in a test tube or elsewhere outside the body.

LAPAROSCOPE: A surgical procedure in which a fiber optic instrument is inserted through the abdominal wall to view the organs.

LH: Luteinizing hormone. A hormone that triggers ovulation.

LMP: Last menstrual period. By convention, pregnancies are dated in weeks, starting from the first day of a woman's last menstrual period. If her menstrual periods are regular and ovulation occurs on day 14 of her cycle, conception takes place about two weeks after her LMP.

LO: Little One.

LO: Left ovary.

LP: Luteal phase. Basically, the two-week wait.

LSP: Low sperm count.

M/C: Miscarriage. The expulsion of a fetus from the womb before it is able to survive independently, especially spontaneously or as the result of an accident.

MEDICATED CYCLES: Uses ovulation induction medication to coordinate the body's timing with the transfer, ensuring preparation for a potential conception.

MEIOSIS: The form of cell division that creates gametes, or sex cells (eggs or sperm). It is a special form of reproduction that results in four next-generation cells, rather than just two, from each cell.

MENOPAUSE: The ceasing of menstruation. The period in a woman's life (typically between 45–50 years of age) when this occurs.

MENSTRUATION: The periodic discharge of the blood-enriched lining of the uterus through the vagina.

MESA: Microsurgical epididymal sperm aspiration. A procedure to retrieve sperm directly from the epididymal tubule in instances when the man has an unfixable blockage.

METFORMIN: A diabetes medicine sometimes used for lowering insulin and blood sugar levels in women with polycystic ovary syndrome (PCOS).

MF: Male factor.

MORPHOLOGY: The size and shape of sperm is one factor examined as part of a semen analysis to evaluate male infertility. Results are reported as the percentage of sperm that appear normal when semen is viewed under a microscope. Normal sperm have an oval head with a long tail. I would really like to know what the other sperm look like, lol!

MOSAICISM: The presence of two different genotypes in an individual that developed from a single fertilized egg. As a result, the individual has two or more genetically different cell lines derived from a single zygote.

MOTILITY: Refers to the movement and swimming of sperm. Poor sperm motility means that sperm do not swim properly, which can lead to male infertility. Poor sperm motility is also known as asthenozoospermia. How do they come up with these words?

MTFHR: Methylene tetrahydrofolate reductase. The rate-limiting enzyme in the methyl cycle plays a role in processing amino acids, the building blocks of proteins.

NIPT: Noninvasive prenatal screening test. This reveals your baby's risk for genetic disorders and chromosomal abnormalities. It also reveals gender.

NT: Nuchal translucency scan. An ultrasound done between eleven and fourteen weeks of pregnancy to test for chromosomal abnormality, usually Down syndrome.

NTD: Neural tube defects. Birth defects of the brain or spinal cord. They happen in about three thousand pregnancies each year in the United States.

OHSS: Ovarian hyperstimulation syndrome. A possible complication from some forms of fertility medication. When too much hormone medication is in your system, it can cause your ovaries to become swollen and painful. Severe OHSS can cause rapid weight gain, abdominal pain, vomiting, and shortness of breath.

OI: Ovulation induction. Fertility treatment that induces ovulation.

OMNITROPE: A form of human growth hormone (HGH) used to treat growth failure in children and adults who lack natural growth hormone, including those with chronic kidney failure, Turner syndrome, short stature at birth with no catch-up growth, and other conditions.

OOCYTE: A cell in an ovary that may undergo meiotic division to form an ovum.

OPK: Ovulation prediction kit. Helps determine the time in the menstrual cycle when getting pregnant is most likely.

OPU: Oocyte pick-up. Procedure to collect eggs from the ovaries (also called EPU).

OT: Ovulation tracking. Fertility treatment that tracks (through blood tests and ultrasounds) someone's menstrual cycle and the best time to procreate.

OV: Oocyte vitrification. One of the techniques used to preserve fertility. It allows a woman's reproductive capacity to be postponed for as long as she wants, with the same possibilities for conception as at the point when the oocytes are vitrified.

OVARIAN CYST: A fluid-filled sac in the ovary. The most common type of ovarian cyst is called a follicular cyst. It results from the growth of a follicle. In some cycles, this follicle grows larger than normal and does not rupture to release the egg.

OVIDREL: An injectable medication used to help with ovulation (egg release) in some fertility regimens. A synthetic LH that is normally produced by the body. Also known as a trigger shot or as recombinant humanized chorionic gonadotropin (hCG).

OVULATION: The release of an egg, or ovum, which may then be fertilized by a sperm cell or dissolved during menstruation. The ovulation process is defined by a period of elevated hormones during the menstrual cycle.

OW: Oocyte warming. Thawing eggs to fertilize.

PCOS: Polycystic ovarian syndrome. A condition in which follicles in a woman's ovaries stall during development and form cysts instead of releasing an egg. Women with PCOS may have infrequent or prolonged menstrual periods or excess male hormone (androgen) levels. The ovaries may develop numerous small collections of fluid (follicles) and fail to regularly release eggs.

PCT: Postcoital test (also known as Sims test, Huhner test, or Sims-Huhner test). A test in the evaluation of infertility. The test examines interaction between sperm and mucus of the cervix.

PESA: Percutaneous epididymal sperm aspiration. A technique used to extract sperm when the man has a blockage of the vas deferens.

PGD: Preimplantation genetic diagnosis. A procedure used prior to implantation to help identify genetic defects within embryos. This serves to prevent certain genetic diseases or disorders from being passed on to the child.

PGS: Preimplantation genetic screening. A test used to determine if genetic or chromosomal disorders are present in embryos produced through IVF.

PICSI: Physiological intracytoplasmic sperm. A technique used in ICSI to help select the healthiest sperm.

PITUITARY GLAND: The major endocrine gland. A pea-sized body attached to the base of the brain. The pituitary is important in controlling growth, development, and the functioning of the other endocrine glands.

PMS: Premenstrual syndrome. Refers to physical and emotional symptoms that occur in the one to two weeks before a woman's period. Symptoms often vary between women and resolve around the start of bleeding. Common symptoms include acne, tender breasts, bloating, feeling tired, irritability, and mood changes. I feel like my "mood changes" last for two weeks.

POAS: Pee on a stick. Taking a pregnancy test.

PRIMORDIAL: In the earliest stage of development.

PROGESTERONE: A steroid hormone released by the corpus luteum that stimulates the uterus to prepare for pregnancy.

PROLACTIN: A hormone released from the anterior pituitary gland that stimulates milk production after childbirth.

RE: Reproductive endocrinologist (fertility specialist). A doctor who has special training in diagnosing and treating disorders of the endocrine system. These disorders include diabetes, infertility, and thyroid, adrenal, and pituitary gland problems.

REPRODUCTIVE SURGERY: Used to correct anatomical abnormalities, remove scarring, and clear blockages in either the man or the woman.

RO: Right ovary.

SA: Sperm/semen analysis (also called seminogram). Evaluates certain characteristics of a male's semen and the sperm contained therein. It is done to help evaluate male fertility, whether for those seeking pregnancy or verifying the success of a vasectomy.

SART: Society for Assisted Reproductive Technologies. Primary organization of professionals dedicated to the practice of ART in the United States.

SD: Sperm donor. See DS (Donor Sperm).

SIS: Saline infusion sonohysterography, or saline ultrasound. A test during which a small volume of saline is inserted into the uterus. This allows the lining of the uterus to be clearly seen on an ultrasound scan.

SIUI: Stimulated IUI. Like IUI, but given medications (FSH) to increase the response of the ovaries to produce a follicle.

SMU: Second morning urine. Is obtained spontaneously after the first morning urine but before noon.

SPERM COUNT: A measure of the number of spermatozoa per ejaculation or per measured amount of semen, used as an indication of a man's fertility. Normal sperm counts range from fifteen million to more than two hundred million sperm per milliliter of semen. You are considered to have a low sperm count if you have fewer than fifteen million sperm per milliliter or fewer than thirty-nine million total sperm per ejaculate. Isn't that like almost unbelievable? That's like quadrillions per person.

STD: Sexually transmitted disease. Any various disease or infection that can be transmitted by direct sexual contact, including those spread chiefly by sexual means and others such as syphilis, gonorrhea, chlamydia, genital herpes, hepatitis B, and AIDS.

SURR: Surrogate. A woman who becomes pregnant, usually by artificial insemination or surgical implantation of a fertilized egg, for the purpose of carrying the fetus to term for another recipient.

TB: Testicular biopsy. A test to remove a small sample of tissue from one or both testicles. The tissue is looked at under a microscope to see if the man is able to father a child.

TD: Treatment day. Refers to what day in the IVF treatment you are.

TESE: Testicular sperm extraction. The process of removing a small portion of tissue from the testicle under local anesthesia and extracting the few viable sperm cells present in that tissue for intracytoplasmic sperm injection (ICSI).

TI: Timed intercourse. You are having sex around the time of ovulation, usually within one or two days of positive ovulation test (or spike in temperature, if you are charting your BBT). Similarly, timed intercourse means having sex every other day around the time of ovulation.

TRIGGER: hCG shot given to induce ovulation.

TROPHECTODERM: Another term for trophoblast.

TROPHOBLASTIC CELLS: Cells forming the outer layer of the blastocyst that provide nutrients to the embryo and develop into a large part of the placenta.

TSH: Thyroid-stimulating hormone. A hormone produced by the pituitary gland at the base of the brain in response to signals from the hypothalamus gland in the brain. Promotes the growth of the thyroid gland in the neck and stimulates it to produce more thyroid hormones.

TTC: Trying to conceive.

TWINGES: Spotting of blood.

UNDESCENDED TESTICLE: A testicle that hasn't moved into its proper position in the bag of skin hanging below the penis (scrotum) before birth. Usually just one testicle is affected, but about 10 percent of the time, both testicles are undescended.

URETHRA: The duct by which urine is conveyed out of the body from the bladder; in male vertebrates, it also conveys semen.

UTERINE LINING: The inner layer of the uterus (womb). The cells that line the womb; anatomically termed the endometrium. This tissue is normally shed monthly in response to the hormonal changes of the menstrual period.

UTERUS: The organ in the lower body of a woman or female mammal where offspring are conceived and in which they gestate before birth; the womb.

VAS DEFERENS: The duct that conveys sperm from the testicle to the urethra.

VZV: Varicella zoster virus. Better known as herpes, chicken pox, or shingles.

WASHED SPERM: A process that separates viable sperm cells from the seminal fluid.

WFP: Wait for period.

WIC: Where in cycle. Referred to when someone is unsure at what day in their menstrual cycle they are and requires a blood test to determine this.

ZIFT: Zygote intrafallopian transfer. Like IVF, but the embryo is inserted into the fallopian tube, not the uterus. The minute the egg is fertilized, it is called a zygote. It spends more time in the body than the lab, so some people feel like the body is a better incubator than a petri dish.

ZONA PELLUCIDA: The thick transparent membrane surrounding a mammalian ovum before implantation.

ZYGOTE: A diploid cell resulting from the fusion of two haploid gametes; a fertilized ovum.

References

Top 100 Fertility Acronyms Decoded. (2014, July 2). Retrieved from https://www.genea.com.au/my-fertility/why-genea/blog/all-blog/july-2014/top-100-fertility-acronyms-decoded

Johnson, T. (2017, January 21). Infertility Drugs. Retrieved from https://www.webmd.com/infertility-and-reproduction/infertility-medications

Ding, K. (2017, March). Fertility Treatments: Your Options at a Glance. *BabyCenter Medical Advisory Board*. Retrieved from https://www.babycenter.com/0_fertility-treatment-your-options-at-a-glance_1228997.bc

Female Fertility Testing (2017, May 16). Retrieved from http://americanpregnancy.org/infertility/female-fertility-testing/

Christiano, D. (2018). Learn About Your Fertility Treatment Options. Retrieved from https://www.parents.com/getting-pregnant/infertility/treatments/guide-to-fertility-methods/

Schneider, Pearson, and Valiente. (2014, November 13). Meet the Men Having Sex with Strangers to Help Them Have Babies. Retrieved from https://www.abcnews.go.com/amp/Lifestyle/meet-men-sex-strangers-babies/story%3fid=26870643

Grunebaum, A. (2018). 2WW Symptoms: Two Week Wait Symptoms. Retrieved from https://www.babymed.com/pregnancy-symptoms/2ww-2-week-wait-symptoms

Padmasekar, M. (2018). Does Taking Supplements Help IVF Patients. Retrieved from https://www.drmalpani.com/articles/taking-supplements-help-ivf-patients

Successful Fertility Treatment: How Much Will It Cost You? (2018). Retrieved from https://www.fertilityauthority.com/articles/successful-fertility-treatment-how-much-will-it-cost-you

Infertility Financing Programs. (2017, November). Retrieved from https://resolve.org/what-are-my-options/making-infertility-affordable/infertility-financing-programs/

Davenport, D. (2018). Books for Children Conceived Through Sperm Donation. Retrieved from https://creatingafamily.org/infertility/suggested-books-for-adults-and-kids/books-children-conceived-sperm-donation/

Fine, E. (2009). Infertility: A Philosophy of Fertility Enhancement. Retrieved from http://fineacupuncture.com/infertility.php

Nemiro, J. (2017). Grading IVF Embryos. Retrieved from
https://www.acfs2000.com/ivf-embryo-grading.html

Embryo Growth is Monitored in the IVF Lab. (2017). Retrieved from
http://ivfplano.com/ivf/embryo-growth/

PGD and IVF - Preimplantation Genetic Diagnosis and In Vitro Fertilization, Pros and
Cons About PGD and PGS. (2017). Retrieved from
https://www.advancedfertility.com/preimplantation-genetic-diagnosis.htm

The Egg Retrieval Process. (2018). Retrieved from
https://extendfertility.com/our-process/the-egg-retrieval

Brighton, L. (2011, December 11). Pregnancy Test Sensitivity List Information.
Retrieved from
https://community.babycenter.com/post/a30635441/pregnancy_test_sensitivity_list_info
rmation

Fowler, A. (2014, April 19). 23 Weird, Common, and Unique Very Early Pregnancy
Symptoms. Retrieved from
https://livelikeyouarerich.com/23-weird-common-and-unique-very-early-pregnancy-
symptoms/

The Procedure. (2018). Retrieved from
https://attainfertility.com/understanding-fertility/treatment-options/iui/the-procedure/

Human Chorionic Gonadotropin (hCG): The Pregnancy Hormone. (2017, August).
Retrieved from
http://americanpregnancy.org/while-pregnant/hcg-levels/

HCG level chart during pregnancy. (2018). Retrieved from
https://www.huggies.com.au/pregnancy/early-stages/symptoms/hcg-levels

Pahuja, M. (2017, July 26). Retrieved from
https://www.insideradiology.com.au/sis/

America's #1 Independent Pharmacy. (2017). Retrieved from
http://mdrusa.com

Rupinta, A. (2018, March 7). Retrieved from
http://abc13.com/family/new-in-vitro-method-could-be-game-changer-for-aspiring-
parents/3187255/

Dubin, A. (2018). Retrieved from
https://www.parents.com/pregnancy/everything-pregnancy/kim-kardashian-had-
placenta-accreta-what-is-that/

Nightlight Christian Adoptions. (2018). Retrieved from
https://www.nightlight.org/

Trying to Conceive and Pregnancy Community. (2013). Retrieved from
http://www.twoweekwait.com

Progyny. (2018). Retrieved from
https://www.fertilityauthority.com

Compassionate Care. (2018) Retrieved from
https://www.fertilitylifelines.com/en_US/home.html

First Steps. (2018). Retrieved from
http://fertilitybydesign.com/

Brizendine, Louann M.D., *The Female Brain* (Morgan Road Books, 2006), 75.

Fett, Rebecca, *It Starts with an Egg: How the Science of Egg Quality Can Help You Get Pregnant Naturally, Prevent Miscarriage, and Improve Your Odds in IVF*, (Franklin Fox Publishing, 2014), 78.

Evans, A. (2014, February 18). All About CoQ10 (and how to get it in your plant-based diet). Retrieved from
https://www.onegreenplanet.org/vegan-food/all-about-coq10-and-how-to-get-it-in-your-plant-based-diet/

Cohen, J. (2018, March 26). 30 Proven Alpha Lipoic Acid Benefits + Side Effects, Dosage. Retrieved from
https://www.selfhacked.com/blog/lipoic-acid/#Natural_Sources

Cohen, J. (2017, October 24). How Vitamin E Can Help Fertility and Pregnancy. Retrieved from
https://www.selfhacked.com/blog/vitamin-e-can-help-fertility-pregnancy/

Can You Get Enough Pycnogenol from Food and Dietary Sources. (2005). Retrieved from
http://www.vitaminstuff.com/qa/antioxidant-pycnogenol-qa-6.html

Antioxidant Resveratrol Found to Promote Healthy Fertility in Women. (2018, February 4). Retrieved from:
https://chronoceuticals.com/antioxidant-resveratrol-found-promote-fertility-women/

The Role of Melatonin in Fertility and conception. (2017). Retrieved from
https://www.chronobiology.com/the-role-of-melatonin-in-fertility-and-conception/

Phillips, K. (2015, January 23). Foods for Sleep, a list of the Best and Worst Foods for Sleep. Retrieve from
http://www.alaskasleep.com/blog/foods-for-sleep-list-best-worst-foods-getting-sleep

Barton-Schuster, D. (2015). Improve Your Fertility with Vitamin C. Retrieved from
http://natural-fertility-info.com/vitamin-c-to-improve-fertility.html

Barton-Schuster, D. (2015). Cinnamon benefits PCOS, Endometriosis, Uterine Fibroids & Menorrhagia. Retrieved from
http://natural-fertility-info.com/cinnamon-benefits-pcos-endometriosis-uterine-fibroids-menorrhagia.html

Rodriguez, H. (2015). Prepare for Conception with a Multivitamin. Retrieved from http://natural-fertility-info.com/multivitamin

Myo-Inositol. (2016, September 15). Retrieved from https://www.allinahealth.org/CCS/doc/Thomson%20Alternative%20Medicine/48/10290.htm

Home Remedies to Help You Conceive. (2015, May 29). Retrieved from https://www.top10homeremedies.com/home-remedies/home-remedies-to-help-you-conceive.html

Peterman, W. (2017, October 13). The Benefits of Taking DHEA. Retrieved from https://www.livestrong.com/article/352307-the-benefits-of-taking-dhea/

If You Want to Avoid Early Aging, get to Know DHEA. (2018). Retrieved from https://bodyecology.com/articles/avoid_early_aging_dhea.php

Jing, J. (2018, January 18). B Complex and Fertility. Retrieved from http://www.cycleharmony.com/remedies/fertility-pregnancy/b-complex-and-fertility

Rodriguez, H. (2015). Are You Getting Enough Calcium to Get Pregnant. Retrieved from http://natural-fertility-info.com/are-you-getting-enough-calcium.html

Rodriguez, H. (2015). Omega 3-6-9, Essential Supplement for Fertility and Pregnancy. Retrieved from http://natural-fertility-info.com/essential-fatty-acid-fertility

Hostile Cervical Mucus and Evening Primrose Oil for Fertility. (2018). Retrieved from https://www.early-pregnancy-tests.com/evening-primrose

Barton-Schuster, D. (2015). Fertility Herbal Tonic: Red Raspberry Leaf. Retrieved from http://natural-fertility-info.com/red-raspberry-leaf.html

Patenaude, C. (2012, June 17). Can Probiotics Influence Fertility? It's conceivable. Retrieved from https://holisticprimarycare.net/topics/topics-a-g/digestive-health/1351-can-probiotics-influence-fertility-its-conceivable.html

You are Not Alone. Resolve Will Help You Connect with the Resources You Need. (2018). Retrieved from https://resolve.org/

Blastocyst embryo grading pictures and photos from IVF, In Vitro Fertilization (2017) Retrieved from https://www.advancedfertility.com/blastocystimages.htm

Journey. "Don't Stop Believin'." Columbia Records, 1981.

Clarkson, K. "Piece by Piece." RCA, 2015.

Isaak, C. "Wicked Games." Reprise, 1990.

A Fine Frenzy. "Almost Lover." Virgin, 2007.

Guns N' Roses. "Patience." Geffen, 1988.

Furler, S. "Unstoppable." Monkey Puzzle & RCA, 2016.

Raitt, B. "I Can't Make You Love Me." Capitol, 1991.

McBride, M. "In My Daughter's Eyes." RCA Nashville, 2003.

Printed in Great Britain
by Amazon